Getting the Therapy, Benefits, and Resources Your Child Needs

A Guide for Parents of Children with Cerebral Palsy and Brain Injury

Richard P. Console, Jr

ISBN-13: 978-0-615-29606-7
ISBN-10: 0-615-29606-8

Richard P. Console Jr. Esq.
One Liberty Place
1650 Market Street 36th Floor
Philadelphia, PA 19103
Toll free: 1-800-208-3494
Website: http://www.childbraininjury.org
Email: info@childbraininjury.org

Lighthouse Media Publishing
Philadelphia, PA 19103

Dedicated to Florence and Danielle

Contents

Part II: Know Your Rights

Part III: Conditions and Treatments: What Does the Future Hold?

Part IV: Education

Part V: Estate Planning

Disclaimer: *This book is not a substitute for professional advice, and does not constitute legal advice or an attorney/client relationship. The information in this book is general, and does not cover the laws of all states. For more information on state-specific laws, as well as legal answers that pertain to your specific circumstances, please seek the services of a qualified and experienced attorney.*

Foreword

In December of 2008 my daughter, Danielle, passed away due to complications of anoxic brain damage.

Danielle was born prematurely. Like most preemies at that age, she had some respiratory issues. But aside from the fact that she was very small and tiny, you almost couldn't tell she was premature. She was a very active baby.

Being premature caused some issues with Danielle's lungs, and she was given a respirator tube to help her breathe. A visiting nurse would come to our home every day to give my daughter the care she needed. It seemed as if Danielle was making great progress. And then, one day, everything changed.

Danielle had an episode about a year after her birth that forever altered the course of her life. My daughter's brain went a long time without oxygen. The result was anoxic brain damage.

Who knows what kind of life Danielle could have had? The brain damage caused Danielle to lose her motor skills and her ability to speak. She also needed a feeding tube, and was completely dependent upon others for her care. She needed a full-time nurse during the time I was at work, and also required physical therapy, occupational therapy, speech therapy, and special medical and adaptive equipment.

One of the hardest things about what happened to Danielle was imagining the child she might have been. Another thing that was very difficult was getting Danielle the care she needed. As a matter of fact, this was a constant struggle. It seemed as if every time I turned around the therapy, benefits, and resources we needed to access were just out of our grasp. Often, the therapies Danielle needed were turned down by the insurance company, and they were too expensive for me to pay for on my own. As a parent, it was incredibly frustrating. But one way or another, I knew I had to figure out a way to get Danielle what she needed. I wanted her to live the best life possible.

One treatment I really wanted Danielle to have was hyperbaric oxygen therapy, which is often referred to as HBOT. HBOT has been shown to be extremely effective for kids with special needs, and I noticed that it helped Danielle. Unfortunately, HBOT is expensive, and my insurance company did not want to pay for the treatment.

It was during a time when I felt my emotions, energy, and finances were quickly depleting that I met the author of this book, Richard Console. Richard is an attorney who does a lot of pro bono work for families who need assistance with appeals. In addition to helping individual kids get the therapies they need, Richard is working to ensure that some of these effective therapies are more widely recognized and more consistently paid for by insurance companies.

If you are the parent of a child with special needs I know the kinds of questions you have, the frustrations you face, and how your biggest goal is to make sure your child lives her best life possible. It's a little more complicated to get our children what they need, and it takes a little more time, effort, and research. But with the right support and direction, it can be done.

Florence O.
Lindenwold, New Jersey

Introduction

Finally a reader-friendly, comprehensive resource book that serves as an instruction manual for parents of children with brain injuries acquired at birth or later in life.

When a child acquires a brain injury, parents are thrust into a devastatingly complicated world involving dilemmas they are totally unprepared to handle. They must learn an entirely new language and become assertive and demanding to get services. Parents are sent home from the hospital with a totally different child then the one they had planned for before the incident. Often one parent must quit their job to stay home to care for the child, which adds financial hardship to an already overwhelmed family. Once the initial shock wears off, most parents are hungry for information on how to help get back the child they had before the accident or incident. Rarely is this information made available by the social workers or medical people involved in the child's care. This book is a lifesaver to parents floundering in a sea of confusion and grief.

It covers legal questions parents may have who are considering a possible lawsuit and helps them evaluate their legal options. This book not only addresses what parents' rights are in the legal, medical, and educational systems, but includes information on the various therapies that may help a child recover from a brain injury including the more unconventional therapies such as Hyperbaric Oxygen Therapy, that most medical professionals would never mention to parents, even though it can improve a child with a brain injury much more effectively than the conventional therapies.

Through his selfless dedication, Rick has produced this amazing resource to help parents. This book is a must read for any parent of a child with a brain injury.

Julie Gordon,
Director of MUMS
National Parent to
Parent Network
Green Bay, Wisconsin

Preface

In the past couple of years I've done a significant amount of pro bono work for parents of kids who have suffered from brain injury or cerebral palsy. Much of this pro bono work has centered around getting these kids the treatment and services they need to live the best, most productive, and most independent life possible.

If you are the parent of a special needs child you know that getting benefits isn't always easy. While identifying the kind of treatment your child needs is fairly simple, figuring out how to pay for those services is quite often difficult. There are lots of complicated issues and questions associated with special needs children. Complicated issues and questions also arise such as:

- Is my child entitled to government benefits?
- What is the procedure to apply for government benefits?
- Are there time limits for applying for state and federal benefits?

- Who pays for my child's care?
- What can I do if the insurance company won't pay for a particular treatment?
- What do I do if the treatment my child's doctor suggests is considered "experimental"?
- How do I file an insurance appeal, and what do I do if that gets turned down?
- How do I make sure my child gets the services she needs at school?
- What are my child's legal rights?
- How do I make sure my child will be taken care of if something happens to me?

Many parents that I meet have already tried to answer these questions on their own, and in doing so have more or less exhausted their time and energy—commodities that most families drained by the stress of caring for a child with special needs are sorely lacking. These issues are complicated, and most parents who try to answer them on their own find themselves in a frustrating jumble of red tape.

I began to compile the answers to some of these complex questions some time ago out of concern for a particular client of mine, Florence O. and her daughter, Danielle. Their story, which you can read about in the foreword of this book, was particularly touching to me. Through my work, I knew there were many other families that were going through the same things that Florence and her daughter were going through. I knew there were many other families that shared their struggles, had the same questions, and were running up against similar walls.

Sadly, Danielle passed away before this book could be published, but it is my hope that the information within will help parents of other special needs kids—parents like Florence—take the first step toward advocating for their children and getting the services and benefits their children so desperately need.

This book is not designed to be a legal guide, nor will it answer all questions of parents of children with special needs. Like your children themselves, each family's situation is unique and will require personalized attention. Rather, this book is intended as a launching pad. It is my hope that it will help as many families as possible by giving them some basic guidance. Any legal information you find in this book is general, and may not apply to all states or to your particular situation. Because state laws are very specific, I suggest that you consult with a carefully chosen attorney in your state to determine the appropriate legal actions based upon your specific circumstances, and the local laws.

It is my sincere hope that this book will give you some rudimentary guidance in resolving the complex issues you are currently facing or may face in the future, whether it may be health insurance, long-term care, special education or government services.

One of my goals in my pro bono work is to work toward getting more recognition for alternative and experimental treatments—treatments like hyperbaric oxygen therapy, that have been proven to really work—so that insurance companies are less likely to deny payment for these treatments. By encouraging, educating, and empowering families of children with special needs, I'm hoping that they will join me in my quest to provide peace of mind and hope for the future for parents of children everywhere.

All kids deserve the chance to live the best lives possible. Sometimes you have to fight hard to give them that chance, but with the right information it can be done.

With warm regards,

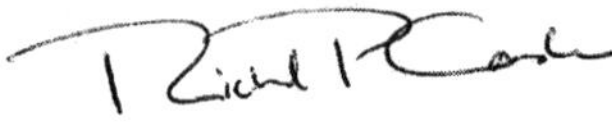

Richard P. Console, Jr., Esq.

Quick Start FAQ List: Getting the Benefits and Therapies Your Child Needs and Deserves

The time following an acquired brain injury may be the most difficult, trying, and frustrating time you'll ever experience in your lifetime. Between coming to terms with the fact that your child's life may be changed, and trying to figure out how to get your child the care he needs, you're bound to encounter one obstacle after another. There is nothing in life that prepares you for this. There are no surefire plans or easy answers. Instead, at a time when you and your child need peace and calm in your life, you'll be assaulted with red tape and headaches.

Like all parents, your number-one goal is to get your child the care she needs, so she can live the best, most productive life possible. We understand. Below are some questions that parents of children with brain injury and cerebral palsy have asked. I chose these particular questions because these and others like them are the kind of questions that parents seem to ask over and over again.

All the answers to these questions are covered in more detail throughout this book. In the meantime, the answers below should put you on the right path to advocate for your child.

Q: Do I need a lawyer, and if so when?

A: The issues and questions that go hand in hand with special needs children are so complex that all parents benefit by engaging an attorney. Because each child's situation is unique, and because state laws vary, there is no one book or resource—including this one—that can effectively give parents the know-how they need to successfully navigate the myriad legal, financial, and educational issues they are going to face. To ensure that your child gets all the services and therapies he needs, your best bet is to hire an attorney who has experience representing children in circumstances like yours, and is familiar with the specific laws in your state (or the state the injury occurred in, if there was an injury involved).

Finding the right attorney is key to ensuring that your child gets what she needs, so the process shouldn't be taken lightly. Before you engage an attorney, you should undertake a rigorous evaluation process. Begin by contacting the State Bar Association for recommendations, and also talk to other parents of kids with special needs to find out whom they have used successfully. Your child's physician or members of her rehabilitation team may also have suggestions. Try regional and national organizations that deal with CP or TBI for recommendations. Narrow your list down to several attorneys, and then interview each one to find the one who has the most experience and suits your particular needs the best. Even if the attorneys you interview don't have the particular expertise you are looking for, chances are they will know someone who does. Engaging the right attorney will maximize the chances of your child getting the benefits he needs—even some benefits you probably aren't aware of.

As far as *when* you should engage an attorney, the answer is ASAP, particularly if your child's cerebral palsy or brain injury was the result of an accident. In addition to there being timing issues when it comes to applying for federal benefits, it's important to get any investigators, engineers, and accident reconstructionists involved early before memories fade and evidence is lost. Many people wait because they are concerned about the costs involved in hiring an attorney. Depending upon your particular situation an attorney may charge a contingency fee (he only collects money if and when you do) or she may charge on an hourly basis. Consultations are generally free, so it's smart to set one up.

If you've already engaged an attorney then congratulations—you have taken the first step to making sure your child gets the benefits and therapies he needs. But if you feel like your current attorney isn't well suited to your situation—if he doesn't have the right experience, or if he doesn't seem committed to your child's case—then it's perfectly acceptable to solicit a second or third, or even a fourth, opinion. The key is to get an attorney you trust to advocate for your child right away. Base your choice on the experience and commitment level of your attorney, as well as whether or not the two of you "click."

Q: My son's doctor has recommended hyperbaric oxygen therapy (HBOT) for his cerebral palsy, and studies show that in many cases it does have a positive effect. But my insurance company has refused to pay for the treatments, saying that HBOT is an "experimental" treatment. They won't budge, even though my doctor says the treatment is needed. Is there a way to challenge this decision, and if so, what is the procedure?

A: Insurance questions rank among the highest percentage of those I get from parents of special needs children. The reason is this: insurance companies will do just about whatever they can to get out of paying your claim. As a matter of fact, there are people employed by your insurance company whose only job is to figure out ways to get around paying claims.

First of all, you want to start by reading your policy. That's because lots of times the answers your insurance company gives you regarding care conflict with what's actually covered in the policy. If you have a hard time getting the insurance company to mail you a complete copy, talk to the human resources department of the policyholder. They should have a complete copy on file.

Once you've received the master policy, go to the section that defines "experimental" treatments. Read it carefully to determine how it relates to the treatment you are requesting.

Next, make a photocopy of this section and bring it to your doctor. When it comes to appealing treatments that have been denied by your insurance company, your doctor is one of your greatest advocates. He will have your child's complete records, and will also be able to explain why, in your child's specific situation, a particular type of treatment is needed.

Your doctor can also point you in the right direction regarding studies and research that show how the denied treatment has helped in the past. The next step requires time, effort, and research on your part, with the goal being to prove that the treatment isn't really experimental. Check out the hospital medical library or do some research on the Internet to prove that the treatment works and is medically necessary.

Once you've gathered all your information regarding the treatment, file the appeal, taking care to follow the guidelines and timelines stipulated by your insurance company. Be sure to get an advocate on your side—whether it's a lawyer or a person from an organization that specializes in advocating for denied claims. There is some good news when it comes to appealing denied claims. When it's done correctly, appealed denials are reversed about 75 percent of the time.

To learn more about dealing with insurance issues, see Part I, "Navigating the System," which begins on page 1.

Q: My daughter was injured in an automobile accident three years ago, and the result was a severe brain injury. We are currently on Medicaid, but are pursuing a third-party claim. We have been told that if we receive a settlement, we'll no longer be eligible for any kind of government aid. We really need those benefits! Is there anything we can do?

A: It is true that receiving a settlement can affect your child's governmental benefits, which often puts parents in a quandary. While the benefits are needed to ensure that the right care is received, these benefits often don't allow the recipient to live above poverty level, let alone provide for everything your child needs. Most families do have to find alternative sources to thoroughly fund their child's care, but no one wants to do so at the cost of losing their government benefits.

Fortunately, your child can keep her government benefits if you set up something called a "Special Needs Trust." A special needs trust is the only kind of device that will allow your child to keep her government benefits while also receiving money from the person or organization that caused her brain injury.

When the special needs trust is drafted, as well as how it is drafted, is really important to its success. For example, you'll want to make sure the trust meets all the necessary Medicaid requirements, and that it's approved by a court before you start receiving any third-party money.

For more information on this subject, see Part V, "Estate Planning," which begins on page 124.

Q: My child has suffered from an anoxic brain injury as the result of a near drowning, and now requires the use of a wheelchair. Our insurance policy will not cover the wheelchair because it falls under the category of "durable medical equipment," which our policy supposedly doesn't cover. What can I do?

A: The first thing you need to do is get your master policy, to ensure that durable medical equipment really isn't covered under your current policy. As I stated before, it's not uncommon for a company to say one thing, only to find out that the policy states something entirely different.

If you find that your policy doesn't cover durable medical equipment, or if you've already exhausted the monies for durable medical equipment on other equipment, all is not lost. It's quite likely that you still have monies available for other benefits. For example, maybe you still have benefits left for outpatient therapy or skilled nursing visits.

How can this help you get your child's wheelchair? You can ask the insurance company to "convert" the benefits that remain into a dollar figure. They then send you a check for this dollar figure, which you are able to use to purchase your child's wheelchair. If your health insurance company refuses to convert funds, you may be able to prove that the company is acting in bad faith.

For more information on converting your health insurance benefits, as well as information on insurance in general, turn to Part I, "Navigating the System," which begins on page 1.

Q: My son has cerebral palsy. I want to make sure that he is taken care of and receives all the treatment he needs in the event of my death. At this point, we do not have enough long-term health insurance to pay for his needs. There are lots of policies out there to consider. How do we choose one?

A: There are basically three levels of care at a nursing home: skilled, intermediate, and custodial. When you are looking at a long-term health plan for an aging adult, custodial care is the most important because this is generally the type of care that most nursing home residents require. People with brain injury and other major injuries, however, usually need intermediate and skilled care as well. Therefore, any policy you consider should have all three levels of care.

The policy should also have a guaranteed renewable clause, which will prevent the insurance company from canceling the policy for any reason, including a change in your child's condition.

Finally, long-term-care policies used to pay only for nursing home care. Today, there are a lot of other services that long-term programs will cover, including transitional living care, home health care, apartment and home living centers, adult day care, community skills care, homemaker services, adult foster care, respite care, and hospice care. It's up to you to determine what your child needs, and to ensure that any policy you choose includes the right components. For more information on long-term insurance, as well as insurance in general, see Part I, "Navigating the System," which begins on page 1.

Q: We are in the process of reviewing my wife's medical records to determine whether negligence during the prenatal or birthing process may have caused our son's cerebral palsy. In the meantime, I heard that the statute of limitations is two years. Is this true?

A: I would have to know more about you, such as which state the possible negligence occurred in, to better answer your question. That's because each state has a different statute of limitations pertaining to minors.

In most states, the statute of limitations kicks in for minors once they reach the age of majority. For example, if the negligence occurred in Pennsylvania, then your son would technically have two years from the time he reached the age of eighteen to submit a claim. In other words, he would be able to submit a claim up until the age of twenty. That being said, this period can be significantly shortened by federal, state, and municipal torte claims, not to mention that it varies from state to state. Your best bet in this type of situation is to contact an attorney ASAP.

You can read more about the statute of limitations in Part I, "Navigating the System," which begins on page 1.

Q: My two-year-old child has cerebral palsy, and is definitely going to need special education. Who is responsible for the services she needs, our insurance company or the school district? Where do we go to make sure she gets what she needs?

A: Under the Individuals with Disabilities Education Act, every disabled child is entitled to a "free appropriate education" that is determined under "due process" procedures. In a nutshell, this means that every child is entitled to the tools and environment necessary for that individual to learn, and it is the school district's responsibility to ensure that your child gets what she needs.

When your child enters school, she will go through a process determined by the Department of Education that will evaluate and classify her. Based on the evaluation and classification, an independent education plan, commonly referred to as an IEP, will be developed by both the school and yourself.

That being said, you don't have to wait until your child is of school age to receive educational benefits. Most children with physical or developmental delays are eligible for early intervention services. Talk to your school district right away about early intervention offerings, and ask what you need to do to access them. To learn more about ensuring your child gets the education she needs, read Part IV, "Education," which begins on page 114.

PART I
Navigating the System

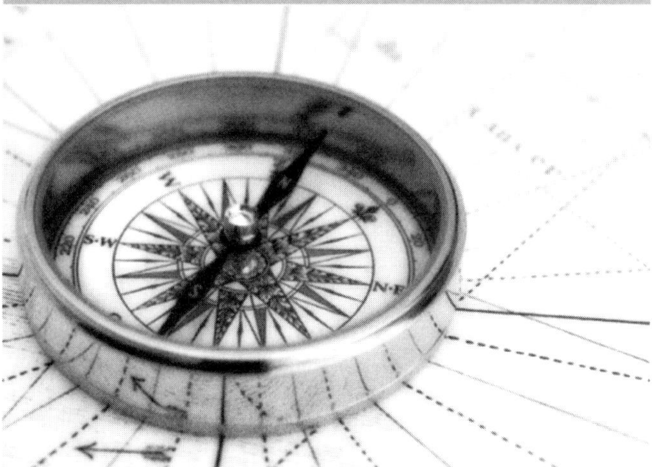

Every parent of a brain-injured child will have to learn how to negotiate "the system" in order for their child to receive what they are entitled to. For the purposes of this section, the system comprises insurance, government benefits, settlements, and estate planning—basically any area you need to navigate on your way to getting your special needs child what he needs and deserves.

The categories in this section are rife with red tape, rules, and regulations that are sometimes very difficult to understand and work around. While it's impossible for the average person to know every nuance and detail associated with the system, knowing some basics should alert you to potential red flags. Know your rights. Be prepared. When you are armed with the right knowledge, you're more likely to get what you want—and need.

The Importance of Advocacy

When it comes to getting your child the care that he or she needs, you'll need to learn how to become an advocate.

That's because you'll have to fight for just about everything that your child needs. If you won't advocate for your child, who will? Insurance companies employ teams of attorneys who are paid to find ways to limit the amount of money that is paid out. They will do whatever they can to find ways to deny important treatments. In addition, government benefits may not be enough, and you may have to wade through lots of complex paperwork and dead-end phone calls to ensure that your child gets the education he is entitled to. One thing is for sure: none of this is going to be easy. However, with the right information—and the right people on your team—you can increase the likelihood of your child getting the treatment she needs. The key lies in educating yourself, and aligning yourself with others who know how to deal with the complex system you'll be battling.

Brain injury support groups are generally organizations that allow brain injury survivors and the loved ones of brain injury survivors to connect and talk to others who have experienced similar ordeals. People in support and advocacy groups share knowledge and experiences, introduce each other to resources, and help each other navigate the many changes they are bound to face as a result of the injury.

While many parents of special needs children put finding a support group on the bottom of their priority list, or plan on finding a support group once things settle down and some sense of normalcy has returned, the early stages are, in fact, the best time to find support and advocacy. Building a support system now will help you prepare for the many issues you are going to face down the road. Remember, because brain injuries behave in an unpredictable manner, you won't know now what the extent of the injury will be, how it will manifest itself, and what specific issues you might encounter later. Having the right people in your corner in a timely manner is key to ensuring that your child gets exactly what he needs and deserves.

Private Insurance

Health care insurance in the United States has changed drastically in the past twenty-five years. Even though many people are covered through government-sponsored insurance such as Medicare and Medicaid, many more people are covered through private, employee-sponsored health plans. When health insurance originally started in the United States, many plans were "indemnity" plans—plans where the patient paid for the service and the insurance company reimbursed the patient. Now this system has changed so the patient is almost entirely omitted from the process. While this may seem like it takes one more hassle off your plate, in effect it makes it difficult for you to be involved in your child's health care decisions.

Most insurance policies are now covered under the

umbrella term "managed care." Under these plans, the patient is required to pay an out-of-pocket co-pay to the provider. The rest of the payment is negotiated between the provider and the insurance company.

Types of Managed Care

Health maintenance organizations, otherwise known as HMOs, are insurance plans that have a predetermined list of medical services that will be covered at 100 percent, but only if the care is given by certain providers within the HMO network. If the service is provided by someone outside the HMO network, no reimbursement will be provided. Additionally, HMOs make the primary care physician the gatekeeper for the child's health care. Each procedure and each specialist must be approved by the primary care physician before the HMO will reimburse it.

Preferred provider organizations, otherwise known as PPOs, are similar to HMOs but provide a higher level of patient autonomy. The patient is free to choose whatever provider or facility they would like, but if the provider or facility is out of the network, the insurance company will pay a reduced reimbursement rate. In addition, the primary care physician is not the gatekeeper to the patient's health care, and patients have more freedom to make their own health care decisions. The downside? PPOs almost always come with higher premiums.

Locating and Understanding Insurance Policies

If your child has had an accident, one of the first things you should do is access your master insurance policies. If these insurance policies are not stored in a safe place in your home, you can get them through your insurance company. Your employer may also have copies of your policy.

It's important to read and understand these policies so you know exactly what your policies cover, as well as what they don't. Depending upon your situation, policies you may want to access include your health insurance policies, automobile insurance policies, and homeowner's insurance policies. These policies can be confusing, so read them carefully. Questions you'll want answered include the following:

- What kind of policy do I have?
- Does my policy have any restrictions regarding doctors, hospitals, or other providers?
- Does my policy have any restrictions to after hours or emergency care?
- What kinds of out-of-pocket costs am I responsible for?
- Am I aware of all potential exclusions or limitations? What are they?

- What kind of procedures do I need to go through to access services?
- What kinds of procedures do I need to go through to access specialty care?
- What is the lifetime limit on this policy?

Determining Cost of Care

While it may seem like the last thing on your mind, one of the parts of dealing with your child's brain injury or cerebral palsy is figuring out how you are going to pay for the care he needs. Emergency treatment is expensive, as are the battery of tests, life-support services, and rehabilitation care associated with brain injury and cerebral palsy. In addition, there's a good chance you won't be working as much as usual, or may even have to take some time off from work. It's important to deal with financial issues at the beginning, so you can concentrate on what really matters—helping your child get well.

Part of navigating your insurance policies is determining a ballpark figure on the cost of your child's care. Will your policies cover the entire cost, or will the amount of your child's care exceed limits? Also, it's important to break the costs down. For example, how much of the total cost is related to emergency care? Tests? Medication? Therapy? This is extremely important since most policies cover different percentages of the cost depending on the types of services used.

We know what you're thinking! This was overwhelming before we threw the math in. Luckily, most hospitals have a financial department that can work with you to figure out the approximate cost of your child's care. The hospital's financial representative may also be able to help you deal with your insurance company and any questions you might have about coverage. They can also help you submit claims, deal with paperwork, and give you suggestions on ways to pay for potentially uncovered costs.

How to Read Your Policy

A health insurance company is required by law to provide a person insured by their plan with a copy of the complete insurance policy, including all addendums and riders. Your request should be made in writing.

Chances are your policy is many pages long, with lots of small print and legal jargon. The first time you read your policy, stick to the basics by focusing on the following:

- Premiums. This is the monthly cost of the health insurance plan that is paid for by you. How much is it?
- Deductibles. This is the amount that must be paid by the policyholder, out of pocket, before benefits can start.

- Co-pay. This is the amount of money the policyholder must pay out of pocket for each visit to the provider. Pay attention, because this amount can vary depending upon whether the policyholder is seeing a primary care physician or is seeking emergency medical treatment.

- Out-of-pocket maximums. This is the maximum amount of money that a policyholder pays. After this has been reached, the health insurance plan must pay for all expenses related to this out-of-pocket maximum.

- Coverage limits. These are similar to out-of-pocket maximums. However, coverage limits apply to the insurance plan and the maximum amount they must cover. After this amount has been reached, all expenses will be the full responsibility of the policyholder.

- Annual and lifetime limits. Some plans have annual coverage limits, while other plans have lifetime coverage limits. With annual limits, coverage will restart at the start of the next calendar year. With lifetime limits, once the coverage limit has been reached the insurance plan will no longer pay for service.

What Benefits Are Available to Your Child?

As you read through your policy you'll begin to realize that there are some components you weren't aware of when you were accessing run-of-the-mill health care. When you are faced with seeking benefits for medical issues such as brain injury or cerebral palsy, coverage becomes significantly more complicated.

Your policy will contain words like these:

- exclusions
- experimental clauses
- definitions
- limitations
- unrealistic treatment guidelines

What do these things mean? Specifically, what do they mean when it comes to your child's coverage?

Basically, these are terms that insurance companies use to deny medical benefits. In many cases, these treatments are necessary for your children. These treatments may include home therapies, medical equipment, rehabilitative care, nursing facilities, or alternative or experimental care.

What are some typical situations in which benefits are denied?

- Certain treatments and services are excluded. These can be necessary treatments and services, such as home care services, skilled nursing care, and durable medical equipment.

- The child's care is not medically necessary. Who decides whether or not your child's treatment is medically necessary? It should be the doctor, right? Not so fast. The insurance company reserves the right to determine, at its own discretion, whether a treatment is medically necessary.

- The medical treatment was not pre-approved. Parents must submit treatments for pre-approval before the insurance company pays for them. If the pre-approval is not submitted for whatever reason, an insurance company reserves the right to deny treatment—even if the treatment is considered necessary.

- The child's care is custodial. Care that is considered "custodial" is care that is not perceived as contributing to the child's gains. If the child has reached a plateau or the insurance company believes the treatment is not contributing to the child's recovery, they may deny treatment.

- If the medical report from the child's doctor does not meet the definitions of the insurance policy. For example, a doctor may prescribe a certain type of assistive technology that does not meet the insurance carrier's definition of durable medical equipment. The carrier can refuse to pay for the technology.

- If the requested treatment is experimental or alternative. For example, very few insurance companies will agree to pay for HBOT, even though its benefits to children with cerebral palsy have been proven.
- The child has reached his or her limit in a particular category. For example, the durable medical equipment benefit is depleted on one item, so no benefit is left for other needed durable medical equipment.

Using Your Bargaining Power

The first thing that parents should do when certain therapies, services, or equipment are denied due to lack of coverage is to ask whether a "conversion" can take place. A conversion is basically when you swap one kind of covered benefit for a benefit that isn't covered. For example, let's say that your child would benefit from Therasuit therapy, but your insurance company doesn't cover it. However, your child does have coverage for thirty skilled nursing visits that aren't, in comparison to the Therasuit, as beneficial to your child's improvement. In effect, you would agree not to use the thirty skilled nursing visits in exchange for the insurance company paying for the Therasuit therapy.

In most cases where a conversion is accepted, the parent has developed a convincing argument that shows how swapping will be beneficial not only to the child, but to the insurance company as well. In the best of situations, the parent finds a downside to the insurance company not agreeing to the conversion; for example, the parent would somehow show how withholding the Therasuit therapy could contribute to more costly medical issues that the insurance company would have to pay for.

When you go the conversion route go right to the top when it comes to whom you deal with at the insurance company. You'll want to deal with someone who has some power to make decisions. Also, be sure to have all your ducks lined up before you make the request. Have all statistics and research regarding the requested therapy on hand, and get testimonials from your child's doctor and medical team.

The Appeals Process

Parents of children with special needs should expect to have to appeal some of the decisions of their insurance company. Parents who challenge denials and have done their homework will have better results than those who aren't well prepared.

If you've already obtained and carefully read your policy as we suggested earlier, you're ahead of most people. The next step is to contact your insurance company and ask them to put their reasons for denying your claim in writing.

Be sure to find out how long you have to appeal your insurance company's decision. In most cases, there are very specific time limits. If you go beyond the specified time limits you'll likely find they are difficult—sometimes impossible—to extend.

The next step is to hire a lawyer or professional insurance advocate to help you wade through the miles of red tape you are bound to encounter. This person will be aware of any potential roadblocks you might face during the appeals process, and will help you navigate them.

Once you file your appeal, you will be notified of your hearing date. Your hearing will be attended by members of a committee, who will hear your case and decide whether or not to grant your appeal. Be sure to gather applicable test results, medical records, and medical reports prior to the date of the hearing. Appeals are more likely to be granted if members of the committee receive paperwork and have a chance to review it prior to the hearing. At this point it's a good idea to ask any treating doctors to clear their schedules for this date. If they are unable to testify in person, you'll need to make arrangements for them to testify by phone.

If there's any research that supports your position, make sure you gather it prior to the hearing. Your lawyer or insurance advocate can tell you what kinds of information the committee is looking for, as well as how to present it.

Your rights under HIPAA become incredibly important during the appeals phase. Check out Part II, "Know Your Rights," which begins on page 58, for more information regarding HIPAA. Make sure you exercise your rights by not allowing your insurance company to have direct access to any medical records or medical staff.

The External Appeals Process

What happens if your appeal is denied? You have the right to another appeal.

However, if you've exhausted the internal appeals process and your benefits are still being denied, it's time to examine your rights to an external appeal. Several state legislators have instituted external reviews in response to the growing issue of HMOs denying benefits. Whether or not you have access to an external appeals process depends upon where you live. In addition, the external appeals process varies from state to state. If you find yourself considering an external appeal, talk to a lawyer or insurance advocate to help you navigate the subtleties of your state's process.

Automobile Insurance

Automobile accidents are one of the leading causes of brain injury every year. Yet in many cases parents realize they don't have enough insurance only after an accident has occurred.

How much automobile insurance an individual should carry depends on a variety of factors, in particular state insurance laws and the driver's own personal and financial situation.

Each state stipulates an insurance minimum coverage. Most states require drivers to carry both bodily injury and property damage coverage so they are covered if someone is hurt in an accident they caused.

How much insurance should you have? As a general rule of thumb, you should carry as much insurance as you can afford, and if you have a high net worth you should carry enough to ensure that you don't stand to lose your assets. If you select limits that are too low, you'll be held responsible for the cost associated with amounts that exceed your limits. In the case of brain injury, this can be financially devastating.

If your child has been brain-injured in an automobile accident there's most likely an automobile liability policy that covered the car she was in. Things you will want to pay attention to include the following:

- The amount of medical coverage the policy allows. This is the amount of money the carrier will pay for your child's injury. Anything beyond this figure is the driver's responsibility. Common limits are $1,000, $2,500, $10,000, $25,000, and $100,000.

- Whether or not you have a limited torte insurance policy. These are available in some states, and stipulate that the driver waives the right to sue for pain and suffering damages unless the injury results in death, serious impairment of body function, or permanent serious disfigurement.
- Whether the policy includes Extraordinary Medical Benefits (EMB) coverage. This kind of optional coverage protects drivers from costs associated with catastrophic injuries. EMB coverage is optional.
- Whether your policy includes underinsured motorist coverage. This type of coverage protects you if your child was injured in an accident caused by another driver who has insufficient liability coverage. As a general rule of thumb, this coverage should be the same amount as the driver's liability coverage.
- Whether your policy includes uninsured motorist coverage. This type of coverage protects you if your child is injured in an accident caused by an uninsured driver. Again, this coverage should be the same amount as the driver's liability coverage.

When Your Child Is Injured in a Different State

If your child is injured in a different state than you live in, it makes sense to talk to your attorney about which state will offer the most medical coverage. For example, state laws in the state you live in might have lower coverage limits than those in the state your child was injured in. Your attorney can carefully consider laws in each state to determine where you will receive the maximum coverage.

Potential Automobile Insurance Problems

There are a variety of potential roadblocks parents might face when trying to ensure that their child's brain injury is covered under the appropriate automobile insurance policy. Some of the more common issues include the following:

1. The definition of "motor vehicle." If your child has been brain-injured in an accident involving a motorcycle, dirt bike, ATV, moped, or snowmobile, your insurance company may try to argue that these things are not officially defined as "motor vehicles" in your policy. Laws will vary from state to state, with some states stipulating that any motor vehicle that is required to be registered falls under the definition of "motor vehicle" for insurance purposes.

2. Signing papers that give away your rights before the full extent of your child's brain injury is determined. If an insurance company gives you a release form or any other document that states you agree to give up your rights, don't sign it! Instead, present it to your attorney, who will give you advice on whether or not signing the document is a good idea. Never feel pressured to sign forms, no matter what an insurance company tells you. It is well within your rights to take the time to read, understand, and consider the implications before you sign any documents.

3. Denial of claims. Any time your claims are denied by your insurance agency, the matter should be discussed with your attorney. Ask the insurance company to put their reason for denying the claim in writing so your attorney can determine whether the denial was wrongful.

4. Slow payment of claims. Slow payment of claims can harm the ability of your child to receive prompt, necessary medical treatment, and may be indicative of bad faith. It is the responsibility of the insurance company to pay all claims in a prompt manner.

Bad Faith

If you believe your insurance company has acted in bad faith, state laws may protect you. Laws pertaining to bad faith vary from state to state.

What kinds of situations constitute bad faith? Any type of situation in which your insurance company denies benefits without good cause, or jeopardizes care by not paying benefits in a timely manner, is considered bad faith.

An insurance company that acts in bad faith is liable for punitive damages, lawyers fees, interests, and court costs. If you feel your insurance company has acted in bad faith, let your insurance advocate or attorney know. She can assess the situation to determine whether damages are likely. In many cases, the act of your attorney writing a letter indicating that you will be seeking damages for bad faith is enough to get the company to correct problems and issues.

Other Sources of Insurance

Depending on where and how the accident that caused the brain injury occurred, other types of insurance might be able to be used. Other common types of insurance that might be accessible in the event of brain injury include the following:

- **School insurance**. If your child becomes injured at school, it's possible the school has insurance coverage to pay for your child's medical bills. If broken equipment, negligent staff, or other avoidable dangers factored into the injury, it's important to contact a lawyer as soon as possible because depending on the state you live in, claims must be filed within a certain amount of time.

- **Homeowner's insurance**. Many homeowner's policies provide benefits that cover a certain amount of medical bills on injuries that occur in the home. It's important to check policies immediately after injury to determine whether there is medical coverage because in most cases notice of the injury and proof of claim needs to be filed within a specified time period.

- **Umbrella/Excess policies**. This is a type of liability insurance policy that takes over where basic liability policies end. An umbrella policy is usually added to the top of a homeowner's or automobile policy, and generally provides coverage of $1 million or more.

- **Third-party claims**. If you believe your child's injury was someone else's fault, or the result of a defective product, or negligence on the part of a third party, you may be entitled to receive benefits under the third party's insurance.

Government Benefits

What happens when the insurance policies run out? Every parent's nightmare is his child sustaining a serious injury. But what's even worse is when there's not enough money to pay for the care your child needs.

Even if you have good insurance, the costs associated with brain injury are so high that eventually even the best of insurance runs out. You can prepare for that time by educating yourself about important government programs.

Medicaid

Medicaid is a type of public health insurance program funded by federal and state money. It's designed for low-income people, as well as people with disabilities who have limited assets. In some states, children with brain injury may also qualify for Medicare services if a certain percentage of their parents' income is going toward medical expenses. A family who has private insurance may still be eligible for Medicaid, and in some cases, where brain injury is particularly debilitating, the child will be accepted into the program regardless of the parents' income.

The Medicaid waiver programs that are available for kids are called Children with Severe Disabilities (CSD) and Home Care for Children with Severe Disability (HC-CSD). Sometimes these are also referred to as the Katie Beckett Waivers.

Every state has different rules regarding Medicaid, in terms of who is eligible, what services are covered, and where services can be received. Types of services Medicaid may cover include medical care, rehabilitation, special equipment and supplies, medical and developmental evaluations, psychological and psychiatric services, and special school services. Certain services that are necessary in the school setting might be covered if they are part of a child's individual education plan, otherwise known as an IEP (for more information on the IEP, see Part IV, which begins on page 114).

The review process for Medicaid can be lengthy, and the application can also be confusing. Parents must fill out something called a "self-determination" form, which asks you to describe your child's disability. The more medical records you include that support your child's diagnosis, the better. Parents who are interested in applying for Medicaid should apply shortly after their child's accident. For more information, contact the U.S. Social Security Association at http://www.ssa.gov/.

Developmental State Disability Program

Every state has programs that are available for children who meet the definition of a developmental disability. Under federal law PL 101-496, a developmental disability is one that is present before the child reaches the age of twenty-two, will last indefinitely, and will result in a need for services over an extended period of time. The disability must cause limitations in at least three of the following areas: self care, learning, economic self sufficiency, communication and understanding of others, mobility, self direction, and independent living.

In order to qualify for services, it's important that your child's diagnosis is correctly defined. You can talk to an attorney, advocate, or knowledgeable doctor about how to best word your child's diagnosis. For parents with children of cerebral palsy, these programs can be particularly helpful.

For more information on your state's developmental disability program, contact the National Association of Developmental Disabilities Council (NADDC), 1234 Massachusetts Ave. NW, Ste. 103, Washington, DC 20005.

Maternal and Child Health

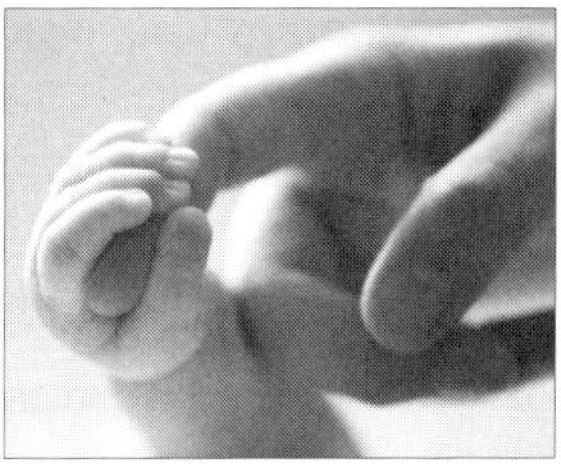

Title V of the Social Security Act allocates a certain amount of money to support kids with special health care needs, including those that result from brain injury. Depending on the state you live in, services might include financial assistance, care coordination, special health care clinics, and information and referrals. For more information contact your state's Department of Health and Human Services.

Social Security

Supplemental Security Income (SSI) is another government benefit available to children with disabilities. In fact, this is the most common income benefit for kids with special needs. However, SSI is not based on how much the parent paid into Social Security. Instead, it is based on a formula that takes both the family's income and the number of people in the family into account.

In order for a child to receive SSI benefits, the SSA must determine that the child is disabled. A child is considered disabled for SSI benefit purposes if his condition results in "marked or severe functional limitations" for at least twelve consecutive months. If a child has a job that is considered "substantial work," the child may not be considered disabled.

Some disabled children will qualify for a different income benefit called Childhood Disability Benefits (CDB). These benefits are usually more generous than SSI benefits, but have certain qualifications that must be met. Children eligible for this benefit must be eighteen years of age, and must have been disabled before the age of twenty-two and remain disabled until their parents retire, become disabled, or die. A child may also qualify if her parents are currently receiving SSDI or SSRI, or if a parent who is insured for Social Security benefits dies. If a child is receiving SSI and Medicaid at the time he qualifies for CDB, he will still be eligible for Medicaid, as long as the child's Medicaid asset limit isn't reached.

Each state coordinates its own Social Security through its district offices. For more general information visit the U.S. Social Security Association website at http://www.ssa.gov/, or reach them by phone at 1.800.772.1213. The world of Social Security benefits can be extremely complex to navigate. If you need help, there are organizations designed to specifically represent or advocate for you. One of those organizations is called the National Organization of Social Security Claimants' Representatives (NOSSCR). For more information check out their website at www.nosscr.org, or give them a call at 1.800.431.2804. Another option is to contact an attorney who specializes in matters related to Social Security benefits. He can also help you figure out your child's eligibility, and can champion the appeals process if needed.

The Appeals Process

If a child is denied SSI or SSDI coverage, both the child and the parents have rights. If you are initially denied coverage, or if your benefits are discontinued, then you have the right to file an appeal. With both SSI and SSDI, there are four levels of appeal, depending on the issue. In order, the levels of appeal are: reconsideration, hearing by an administrative law judge, Appeals Council review, and federal court. Timing is of great importance in filing an appeal. An individual must file an appeal within sixty days of receiving the letter from the Social Security Administration. If an appeal is not filed within sixty days, the individual will more than likely lose the right to appeal, which may permanently close the door on receiving SSI benefits. The request for an appeal must be in writing, and the individual has the right to have legal representation.

Child Health Insurance Program

The Child Health Insurance Program (CHIP) was first introduced by Congress in 1997, and is designed to increase the eligibility for state-sponsored health insurance. The program gives more uninsured kids access to health insurance, by offering it to children of low or moderate income families who have high medical bills, children who are not eligible for Medicaid, and children who aren't covered by other plans.

Eligibility requirements for CHIP are decided on a state-by-state basis, and eligibility requirements are always changing. The rules are different in each state as well, with some states requiring that families contribute up to 5 percent of their income to co-payments, deductibles, and premiums. Contact your particular state for more information.

Other Sources of Funding

In many cases, parents of special needs children need to consider other sources of funding when it comes to paying for the care their child needs. Parents without adequate insurance policies, for example, may find that the government benefits their child is eligible for just don't cover all the bases. Before your child sustained her brain injury or was diagnosed with cerebral palsy you knew there would be normal expenses associated with your child—expenses like food and shelter, clothing, summer camps and hobbies, and other costs associated with growing children. But you probably never dreamed you would have to pay for things like rehabilitative care, adaptive equipment, medication, and specialized housing modifications. When you add these things up, they can be unbelievably staggering.

In many cases the community steps in to ensure that some of the financial burden is taken off the parents. Churches and charitable organizations may hold fund-raisers or have some finances set aside for these types of situations. As a parent it may be difficult to find the time to organize fund-raisers. Luckily, family and friends have been clamoring for a way to help, and this is a great way to get them involved.

National Transplant Assistance Fund and Catastrophic Injury Program

A terrific organization parents of kids with special needs should get to know is the National Transplant Assistance Fund and Catastrophic Injury Program (NTAF). The program's sole mission is to help families organize and launch fund-raising campaigns designed to be used for uninsured medical expenses related to catastrophic injury. The program allows funds to be collected for your child, and then released as needed. This is also a perfect program to look into if your child needs access to an alternative treatment not covered by your insurance, such as HBOT. For more information on this program, contact NTAF at 1.800.642.8399, or visit their website at www.transplantfund.org.

Relief Funds

Several states have enacted legislation to establish Catastrophic Illness in Children Relief Funds, which are designed to help families with the excessive financial burdens that go hand-in-hand with injuries and illnesses such as brain injury and cerebral palsy. These programs are designed to help with expenses that are not covered by private insurers, federal or state health benefits, or another financial source. To find out if your state has a Catastrophic Illness in Children Relief Fund, contact your state government.

Crime Victim Compensation Fund

If your child has been injured as the result of a crime, she may be eligible for funds from your state's Crime Victim Compensation Board. To determine eligibility as well as your state's particular offerings, log on to the National Association of Crime Victim Compensation Board's website, www.nacvcb.org.

Settlements

If your child was brain-injured as a result of someone's negligence, a defective product, or something else that can be construed as misconduct or failure to act, then a personal injury claim is another potential way to fund your child's care. As it's been stated before, one of the biggest issues that parents of brain-injured children will face is how to pay for past, current, and future medical care. A personal injury settlement can insure that the person or entity responsible for your child's accident takes financial responsibility for it.

Since most personal injury attorneys don't charge money to review your case, it certainly doesn't hurt to have your child's situation reviewed. The list below is only a partial list of situations in which a personal injury claim should be considered, and is by no means exhaustive. Have an attorney assess your specific situation.

Automobile Accidents

When your child is injured as the result of some other driver's negligence, the accident should be investigated. The most commons sources of recovery in automobile accidents are against the insurance company of the driver who caused the accident. It's important the parent isn't bullied by the driver's insurance company into taking the first settlement offered because this can result in an amount that doesn't even begin to cover the child's care. If an insurance company asks you to sign any kind of paper waiving your rights or agreeing to a settlement sum they have arrived at, don't sign! Your attorney can handle this matter from start to finish, will ensure the process is handled according to the laws of your specific state, and will negotiate an amount that will get your child the care she needs.

Automobile-related Defects

Lots of brain injuries could be completely avoided or significantly minimized if the automobile the child was riding in was correctly designed. We've all heard the stories of tire blowouts, crushed roofs, poorly designed seat belts, and collapsing seat backs that have caused tragic accidents and even death to passengers. Other defects include those related to braking, steering, and mistakes that cause the car to operate in a dangerous manner.

It is the job of the automobile manufacturer to provide adequately designed safety features to counteract the dangers that a person might encounter while driving or riding in a car. This has resulted in a legal theory called "crashworthiness." If a vehicle is not "crashworthy"—if it has certain design defects or lacks safety features necessary to protect a driver or passenger in the event of an accident—then the manufacturer may be liable for the injuries sustained in the accident.

Here's an example: Let's imagine that a car is rear-ended, and the driver's seat collapses into the back seat, causing a significant head injury to the child seated behind the driver. It would be determined that this vehicle was not "crashworthy."

It's extremely important that the vehicle is not destroyed before a proper and thorough investigation is completed. In many cases, the insurance company carts the vehicle away before anyone has the chance to properly examine it. By the time you realize the car is an important piece of evidence, it's been destroyed. If your car must be towed, be sure whomever takes it away is advised not to destroy it. Common safety hazards and defects that have resulted in settlements include the following examples:

- **Seat belts**. This would include improperly designed or defective rear lap belts, shoulder-only belts, belts with excessive slack, door-mounted belts that have not been retrofitted or recalled, and lap-only seat belts that have not been retrofitted or recalled.

- **Seat backs**. Seat backs should be designed so they can withstand a rear impact. Seat backs that collapse can cause tragic injuries for both the driver and the passenger of the vehicle.

- **Head restraints**. Head restraints that aren't properly designed can cause severe spinal cord and head injuries resulting from rear-end collisions.

- **Airbags**. Airbags are a great safety feature that have saved countless lives, but the tremendous force they exude can cause serious injury or even death when children are involved. Child seats should never be placed in the front seat, and children who do not meet a certain height requirement should ride in the back. Many of today's late-model vehicles have systems that automatically turn front seat airbags off if a person under a certain weight is sitting in the passenger-side front seat, but these should not necessarily be trusted.

- **Child safety seats**. While these seats are designed to protect children in the event of an accident, tragically there have been defective and poorly designed child safety seats that have resulted in injuries and fatalities. Common issues include belt fasteners that don't hold, belts that are too loose, seats that have cracked or shattered upon impact, seats with excessive incline, buckles that come open, and seats with choking hazards.

- **Rollovers**. Rollovers are one of the most common causes of head injury that result from an automobile accident, and are most common with SUVs and other vehicles with a high center of gravity. A rollover is caused by poor design that causes the vehicle to tip over at certain speeds and when going around corners.

- **Roof collapses**. In many situations where rollovers occur, it is roof collapse that causes the head injury. While it would cost very little per vehicle for manufacturers to amend their designs and make their roofs stronger, there is no legislation that currently mandates this. However, there are several advocacy groups that are calling for more stringent requirements when it comes to roof strength.

- **Side impact**. The government currently has side impact standards that every car must pass, but organizations such as the Insurance Institute for Highway Safety, a non-profit organization financed by insurance companies, is trying to get manufacturers to redesign cars so that passengers are safer during side impact collisions.

- **Tire blowouts**. Defective tires, as well as worn and overused tires, can cause tread separation, crashes, and rollovers.

Highway Hazards

Unsafe roadways can also cause accidents that lead to brain injury. In these cases the municipality where the accident occurred may be liable for your child's head injury. It's extremely important to reconstruct the events that led up to the accident as soon as possible after it occurred. If a highway hazard played any part in the accident, it's best if it's identified sooner rather than later. In addition, most states have laws that stipulate the time frame in which a municipality must be notified that it may be sued. Common highway hazards include the following:

- Poor road design
- Poor location of telephone poles
- Improper lighting
- Improper roadway drainage, leading to slippery and icy roads
- Poor maintenance
- Lack of medial barriers
- Lack of warnings and road signs that alert the driver to roadway dangers

Recreational Injuries

Recreational injuries are a common cause of brain injury, especially in children. Common recreational injuries that cause brain injury in children are ATV accidents, swimming pool accidents, recreation-related injuries, and playground accidents. Many times, parents don't seek damages from responsible parties because they believe the accident was actually their fault. However, in many cases this just isn't true. A careful review of your child's accident can determine whether or not someone else is at fault for your child's brain injury.

- **ATV Accidents**. The number of ATV-related emergency room visits continues to grow, with more than half of those sustaining fatal and serious injuries under the age of sixteen. In 2005, the Consumer Product Safety Commission published a report that showed that ATV-related deaths rose from 29 in 1982 to 470 in 2004. Injuries during the same time period rose to a high of 136,100. The Consumer Product Safety Commission has held many hearings on the dangers of ATVs, resulting in unstable three-wheeled models being taken off the market. In addition, several advocacy groups have asked that ATV sales to children be prohibited. Unfortunately, many ATV makers continue to market their vehicle to the younger set, resulting in serious injuries.
- **Swimming Pool Accidents**. Swimming pools have resulted in many serious injuries in children,

specifically anoxic brain injury. Anoxic brain injury results from the brain not getting enough oxygen, and is common in situations in which near drowning occurs. According to the National Safety Council, close to 2,500 children are treated each year in hospital emergency rooms for pool-related injuries, mostly to the spine and head. Swimming pools should have appropriate safety gates and locks, as well as warnings on the pool and in the pool's literature that warn the parents of dangers and instruct them in safety measures. Objects that attract children—such as toys—should be kept out of the pool area, and all water should be drained from pools and spas when not in use because children can drown in as little as two inches of water. Lifeguards, caretakers, and homeowners should know CPR because without prompt administration the child is in danger of suffering an anoxic brain injury. Finally, signs should be posted that warn swimmers from diving into shallow water. Inappropriately placed and designed diving boards can also cause accidents. Parents of children who have suffered serious injuries as a result of diving board accidents should not assume it "was just an accident," but should investigate their particular circumstance to determine if the accident was caused by lack of warning, poor design, or unsafe conditions.

- **Trampoline Accidents.** Trampolines are supposed to be fun, but you have to stop and wonder exactly how fun they really are when you consider the serious injury that frequently results from them. In addition to broken bones and other minor accidents, trampolines are one of the leading causes of brain injury among children. As a matter of fact, according to the Association of Orthopedic Surgeons, 186,405 kids under the age of fourteen are injured on trampolines every year in the United States. Trampolines should never be used by children without adult supervision, and should always be placed on even ground in well-lit areas. The landing areas, as well as supporting bars and strings, should be padded. While netting may be used to reduce the incidence of injury, it should never be substituted for adult supervision. It's important that only one child use the trampoline at a time (many head injuries result from collisions), and flips and other risky tricks should be discouraged.
- **Playground Accidents.** No parent likes to have her child's playground fun curtailed by an emergency room visit. Unfortunately, according to the Centers for Disease Control, more than 200,000 children under the age of fourteen are treated in the emergency room every

year for playground-related accidents. Some of these accidents result in brain injury, most of which are short falls to inappropriate playground surfaces. Defectively designed equipment such as slides, swings, climbing walls, and merry-go-rounds can also cause serious injury. Public and private playgrounds should be age-appropriate, should have non-defective equipment in good repair, should have a safe surface below the equipment, and should be appropriately supervised when minor children are present.

- **Attractive Nuisance Accidents**. An "attractive nuisance" is described as anything on a property which may attract minors and is dangerous to them. Examples are trampolines, swing sets, and unfenced swimming pools. Municipalities, homeowners, and businesses are responsible for taking measures to ensure that children don't have access to any attractive nuisances located on their property.

- **Slips and Falls**. If your child has suffered a brain injury as a result of a slip and fall, it's very important to find out why. Even if nothing in particular stands out at the time, it's important to get photographs of the place in which your child slipped or fell. If there was a foreign substance on the floor such as oil, grease, water, or some other kind of liquid, statements from any witnesses who saw the accident should be taken, and the shoes of the child should be preserved in a plastic bag. Improperly designed stairways, hallways, and railings that aren't up to code, as well as floors that violate mandated standards of friction, can also cause slips and falls that lead to brain injury.

- **Alcohol-related Claims**. If your child's brain injury was the result of an accident with a drunk driver, the circumstances may allow you to file something called a "dram shop" claim. A dram shop claim is a claim brought against a restaurant or bar that served alcoholic beverages to a person who showed signs of being intoxicated. In these situations toxicology and blood alcohol reports, as well as reports from witnesses, are key. In many states a bar or restaurant that serves alcohol to a minor who injures himself may also have a suit brought against them. Finally, some states hold the host of a party liable for any injuries that result from them allowing alcohol to be consumed at any party or gathering they are hosting. For example, a person throwing a wedding with an open bar may be liable for injuries that result from one of the guests causing an accident resulting from intoxication. Again, state laws differ, so check with your attorney regarding potential liability claims associated with alcohol.

Defective Product Claims

If your child's brain injury is the result of a defective or dangerous product, the manufacturer of that product may be liable. Manufacturers of baby walkers, toys, helmets, garage door openers, automatic car windows, and window screens have all been held responsible for head injuries to children.

- **Baby walkers**. More than 8,000 children were treated for injuries related to baby walkers in 2000. About 76 percent of babies under the age of fifteen months that are injured in baby-walker-related accidents fall down stairs, while 12 percent tip over. Of those that fall down stairs, a significant portion sustain some kind of head injury and require hospitalization. As of 1997, all baby walkers made in the United States must be wider than a standard doorway, and must also be equipped with a braking feature that stops the walker at the edge of a step.
- **Toys**. Toys that are choking hazards are the leading cause of anoxic brain damage in young children. Current federal legislation prevents toys with small parts being marketed to children

under the age of three, and warning labels must state the specific reason why the toy is a choking hazard. Latex balloons must also carry a choking warning for kids under the age of eight.

- **Helmets**. Protective helmets are part of the sports equipment for sports such as hockey and football, but are also recommended for activities like horseback riding, bike riding, rollerblading, and skateboarding. Many states also have helmet laws when it comes to ATV riding, as well. While wearing a helmet has significantly cut down on sports-related head injuries—depending upon what statistics you access, up to 85 percent—cases have been brought against helmet manufacturers who have made and sold helmets that have failed to protect their wearer. If your child has sustained a brain injury while wearing a helmet, it's possible the helmet was in some way defective. Parents should make sure that any helmet involved in a brain injury is examined by an expert to determine its strength and durability, whether it should have prevented the injury, and whether it is defective.

- **Window screens**. Every year about 5,000 children fall out of windows. About 28 percent of those falls result in hospital stays. While window screens are not safety devices, all windows that are five feet or more above the ground should have window screens installed that can't be easily pushed out by the weight of the child. In addition, multi-level buildings should be outfitted with window guards, window locks, or wedges that prevent the window from opening too much. Apartment owners, business owners, and screen manufacturers may be liable in the following circumstances:

- Window screens that pop out easily are installed in unguarded windows.
- Window screens are not present.
- Broken window screens are not replaced.
- "Wedges" that prevent windows from opening more than three to five inches were not properly installed.
- Clips holding the screen came loose.

Building codes vary from municipality to municipality, but are important to understand in any situation in which a child falls from a window. You'll have to navigate the often complex building codes of your municipality to determine whether someone else is at fault for your child's accident. Screens should also be saved and examined, and pictures of the window should be taken as evidence.

- **Garage door openers**. Despite advances in the design of automatic garage door openers, children continue to be hurt and killed by them every year. Since 1974, 85 children have either died or sustained permanent brain injury as the result of an accident involving an automatic garage door opener. Most of these accidents are the result of the child being pinned under a door that doesn't reverse. Current Underwriter Laboratory standards call for all garage door openers to be equipped with sensors that cause them to automatically reverse when they come into contact with an object other than the floor, but all too often these systems fail. As a matter of fact, one evaluation of fifty different garage door openers done by the American Academy of Pediatrics showed that 40 percent failed to reverse when they encountered a child-sized mannequin.
- **Power car windows**. The National Highway Traffic Safety Administration says that about 500 people are injured by power car windows every year, most of whom are children younger than fifteen. Of those, one or two die. The injury often occurs as a result of the child putting pressure—through kneeling or leaning—on the toggle or rocker switches that control the windows. The federal government is requiring all manufacturers to install lever switches that

don't respond to unintentional pressure, in all vehicles by October 1, 2010. Advocates of child safety have asked that vehicle manufacturers also install automatic reverse windows in all vehicles. The result is the Gulbransen Act, which was signed by congress in February 2008. This act asks the National Highway Traffic Safety Administration (NHTSA) to mandate automatic reverse windows under the car safety act.

Birth-related Injuries

Unfortunately, medical negligence is responsible for a portion of birth-related brain injuries. If it is determined that medical negligence is the cause of your child's brain injury or cerebral palsy, you may be entitled to financial benefits that cover the cost of your child's needs and care. Medical negligence that results in brain injury or cerebral palsy can occur during pregnancy or during delivery.

Birth-related brain injuries are most often caused by lack of oxygen to the brain. While physicians are trained to notice the signs of cerebral palsy not all do, and this can lead to further brain damage.

Birth-related brain injury can be caused by a number of factors, including but not limited to improper monitoring during pregnancy, failure to screen or treat infection in the mother or child, misdiagnosis of labor, electronic fetal monitoring, premature rupture of membrane, placenta abnormalities, improper administration or dosage of labor-inducing drugs, and cesarean section delays.

If your child is born with a brain injury it's important to rule out medical malpractice as a cause. This is not a determination that's possible for the average parent to make. If your child has a brain injury at birth, be sure to discuss your situation with a medical team as well as an experienced brain injury lawyer. He or she can assess your particular situation and determine whether medical malpractice played a part in your child's brain injury.

Statutes of Limitations

Statutes of limitations for adults vary from state to state, but in most states the injured party must file a suit against the liable party or parties by two or three years following the injury. There are some exceptions to the statutes of limitations, depending on the state you live in.

However, the statute of limitations is *not* the same for adults and minors. In most states (but not all), including Pennsylvania, the statute of limitations for minors does not start ticking until that minor has reached eighteen years of age.

Here's an example. Let's say that Alice, age two, suffers anoxic brain injury as the result of a choking incident caused by a defective and improperly labeled toy.

Alice lives in Pennsylvania, where the statute of limitations for adults is two years. While Alice's parents may, *they do not have to* maintain a claim of action or file a suit within a two-year time frame. Instead, Alice and her parents will have until she reaches the age of twenty—eighteen years—to file a claim.

The best time to file a claim will depend on your child's particular circumstances. Because the extent of a child's brain injury is often not known for some years, in some situations it might make sense to wait, if possible. However, it's really important to stress that the statute of limitations can be shortened by federal, state, and municipal torte claims and issues. Because the statute of limitations varies from state to state, it's imperative that you understand them, and discuss them with your attorney.

Leverage

What happens if your child is injured as the result of someone's negligence, but needs expensive care before a settlement is agreed upon?

In many cases, particularly in cases where little or no medical insurance is available to the injured party, something called "leverage" can be used.

What is leverage? Leverage is when a medical facility that can meet your child's needs furnishes care to your child under the agreement that costs will be covered out of the proceeds of a lawsuit. Leverage can be used when there is little or no insurance, when private insurance is involved, and when government benefits are involved.

Here's an example: Let's say that a four-year-old child suffers a brain injury as a result of a car accident in which a defective driver's seat collapses into the child's space. The child's parents file a lawsuit against the manufacturer of the car with the defective seats. In the meantime, the best rehabilitation center for your child won't accept him, due to insufficient insurance. In many cases, the facility will be willing to entertain the concept of leverage. If the rehab facility agrees to the concept of leverage, it will treat the child with the understanding that all costs associated with the child's medical treatment will be reimbursed to the facility out of the lawsuit proceeds.

Types of Settlements

There are two basic types of settlements—structured settlements and lump sum settlements. In addition to making sure your child is awarded a suitable benefit considering her circumstances, your attorney can also tell which kind of settlement makes the most sense for you.

Lump Sum Settlement

Quite simply, a lump sum settlement is a settlement received in one cash payment. The money from this payment can be used to pay for past, current, and future medical costs.

Structured Settlement

A structured payment is paid out in installments, throughout the life of the child. In a nutshell, an insurance company that specializes in defendant liability buys an insurance annuity, which then pays the child a certain amount of specified benefits. The money is usually managed by a bank or other qualified entity, and because a specified amount is guaranteed to come during certain intervals, it allows the injured party a certain peace of mind concerning the payment of medical costs. On the other hand, there is no flexibility with a structured payment—once the terms are set they can't be changed—and you won't have the ability to do your own investing.

Generally, several proposals will be developed before a structured settlement is agreed upon. It's up to your attorney to review all proposals and determine which one best suits your needs according to potential future medical costs, as well as cost of living increases and inflation.

Subrogation Rights

If you receive a settlement from a third party, the insurance company or other entity that paid for your child's care has the right to recover what they paid for the cost of medical care. These rights are called "subrogation rights." Per federal law the government must also be repaid a certain percentage of money spent on the medical care of a person who later receives a settlement. In addition, people on public assistance are usually required to sign something called a "subrogation form," in which it is agreed that some of the funds will be repaid if the injured party receives a settlement.

When it comes to subrogation rights of medical costs associated with minors who have sustained a brain injury, things can quickly become more complicated. Because of the life expectancy of children and the high costs associated with children's brain injuries, it should be determined by a court how much an insurance company or government agency should be reimbursed. This figure should be based on the estimated amount of time the child will need care and the amount of cost associated with that care, balanced with the amount of money received in the lawsuit and the amount of money paid by the insurance company or government agency.

When You Need a Lawyer

When is it necessary for the parents of a brain-injured child to seek the help of a lawyer? The easy answer is "right away." Now, some of you might be thinking that this is an inappropriate time to be thinking about lawyers because you want to focus on your child getting well. But you'll be more likely to get your child the therapies and benefits she needs to get well if you involve a professional who really knows the ins and outs of the system.

There are lots of reasons why it makes sense for parents of kids with special needs to contact a lawyer. Parents of kids with special needs will need advice on guardianship, private and governmental health benefits, special education benefits, estate planning, and paying for future medical care. They will need an advocate when insurance claims are invariably turned down, and they will need someone on their side to essentially ensure that their kids get the benefits they need.

The sooner the parent seeks advice, the better. That's because in addition to answering legal questions, an attorney who specializes in working with families of special needs children can save you lots of time and money by telling you how best to access the necessary support and services, and can make the road to getting those needed services much smoother. An attorney who specializes in brain-injured children can help you slash through the red tape and navigate the mounds of complex paperwork so your child gets the appropriate care.

An attorney can also help you determine if your child's injury is the fault of another. If you are like a lot of parents of kids who have been injured, you may feel responsible even if it's not your fault. An attorney can tell you whether your child's injury was possibly the result of someone else's negligence. This determination is extremely important, because it can open up additional avenues of funding for your child's therapies and benefits.

When it comes to choosing an attorney, be sure to seek the services of one who has lots of experience dealing with the legal issues associated specifically with children who have cerebral palsy or brain injury. Finding the right attorney is imperative, so do your homework. For a list of attorneys who specialize in this kind of work, get referrals from:

- Your State Bar Association
- Support groups
- National or regional CP or TBI organizations
- Parents of other kids with special needs
- Doctors and specialists on your child's therapy team
- Other attorneys

Once you have a list of qualified attorneys in hand, it's time to narrow it down. Interview potential attorneys face-to-face, and ask questions like:

- How many other families with special needs children with situations similar to mine have you represented in the past?
- Are you currently representing any families with special needs children?

- Do you have any involvement with CP or TBI associations? If so, what is your relationship with them?
- What kinds of advocacy work are you involved in?
- What are some of the results you've gotten for families like mine? (Be sure to ask for specific examples.)
- Do you have the time and resources to take on my case?
- Will you be fully committed to my case?
- What is your opinion on my case?
- When it comes to paying for your services, what are my options?

One of the reasons people hesitate to seek out an attorney is the perceived cost involved. Parents of kids with special needs know that most of their money is going to be spent on their child's medical care, and are hesitant to allocate funds to legal matters. That's a valid concern. However, when it comes to personal injury claims, lawyers use something called a contingent fee agreement. This means the lawyer is paid a percentage of the funds that result from a settlement or lawsuit *only* if the case is won. If the case is not won, the client does not pay the lawyer.

When it comes to issues surrounding guardianship, insurance and benefits, and estate planning, most lawyers charge an hourly fee. However, when parents of special needs children work with an attorney they are much more likely to receive the short- and long-term benefits available to their child—and that can save them a ton of money in the long run. Eligibility requirements are constantly changing, and it's almost impossible for the average person to keep up with them. An experienced attorney can evaluate your case and can tell you what kinds of benefits your child is entitled to, as well as the fastest way to get them.

PART II
Know Your Rights

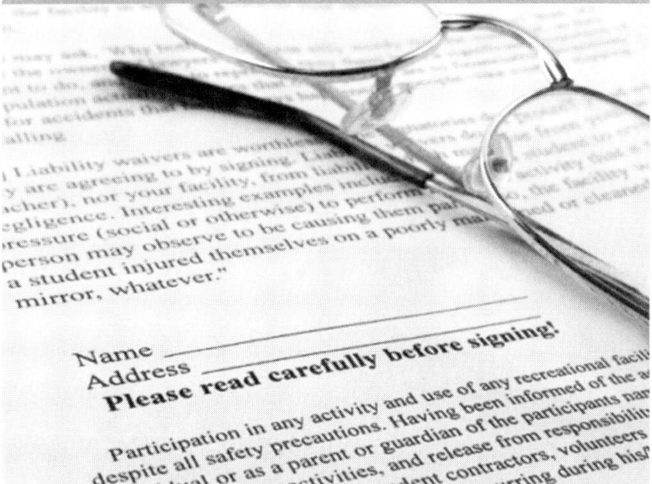

In addition to understanding the many different vehicles that will help get your child the therapies and benefits she needs, you'll also need to be acutely aware of your child's rights as a patient, and your rights as that child's parent.

The time immediately following your child's injury will be spent in the hospital, where you'll be working with doctors and a medical team to determine the extent of the injury and what that means for the future, as well as figuring out a course of action designed to ensure that your child returns to the maximum functionality possible. It goes without saying that the doctors, nurses, and other professionals on your medical team have the best interests of your child at heart. However, in order to ensure that your child receives the best care possible—both now and in the future—it's important that you are well aware of the rights of both you and your child. Not being fully aware of your rights can result in tragic consequences—including your child not getting all the benefits that he needs.

During a time that's so fraught with emotion, it's

tough to pay attention to all the paperwork that's put in front of you. And sometimes it's almost impossible to discern what information you should give to an insurance company, and what information you shouldn't. Most parents are so concerned with the well-being of their children that they haven't a clue what they are signing, or what they are allowing. It's important to emphasize here, however, that being aware of your rights goes hand-in-hand with the care your child will receive. Be attentive, and be careful. Below are things that every parent of a brain-injured child should be aware of.

Consent

One of the many initial issues that parents must concern themselves with is consent. Consent ensures that your child receives timely and necessary treatment. There are three kinds of consent: informed consent, actual consent, and implied consent.

Informed Consent

The term "informed consent" is thrown around very loosely in the medical profession. The first thing we want parents who are reading this book to understand is that informed consent is *not* a medical term. Rather, it's a legal doctrine based upon certain rights that are granted to a patient by law.

When it comes to making health care decisions related to your child, it's important that you are informed of your options. Through the doctrine of informed consent, health care providers are obligated to disclose certain information to the patient regarding their medical diagnosis, the treatment options available, and any risks associated with those options. A failure to disclose this information could adversely affect the patient because the patient would be making an uninformed decision that could potentially lead to serious repercussions.

Competence is important in determining who makes decisions regarding informed consent. When an adult is deemed "incompetent," for example, due to mental disability, the medical professional may have the authority to determine what is best in terms of care. However, when a child is the patient, the child is automatically considered incompetent because it is thought that the child is not able to fully grasp the facts of the situation and is therefore unable to make informed decisions. In these cases, it is the provider's duty to fully inform the parents or guardian of the condition, as well as of available treatment options, so the parents can make an informed decision for the child.

Actual Consent

Once the medical professional has explained the potential outcome and risks of the procedure, as well as the risks and outcomes of possible alternative treatments, the parent or guardian of the child will be asked to sign a consent form that gives permission for the medical team to perform the procedure. This is called actual consent.

Implied Consent

But what happens if you aren't immediately available at the time of your child's injury? Can the medical team treat your child without your consent?

The answer is yes. The legal doctrine of implied consent was developed specifically for situations in which an individual is unable to grant actual consent. Any time there's an emergency, the patient's consent is considered implied.

An emergency is basically defined as any situation that is life threatening and requires immediate attention. Let's say, for example, that your child is in a car accident and sustains serious injuries. No one in the car—neither the driver nor any of the other passengers—is the guardian of the child. You and your spouse cannot be reached. What happens?

Under the doctrine of implied consent, your child will be treated immediately at the scene by paramedics or EMTs, then transported to the hospital where additional emergency treatment will take place. There's no specific time frame that defines an emergency. Instead, an emergency lasts as long as it takes to stabilize the child—as little as a couple of hours or as long as several weeks. Doctors and other medical professionals are allowed to give life-sustaining care to the child during this time.

Once the child is stabilized and his life is no longer in immediate danger, informed consent will be necessary for any additional procedures. While doctors may make recommendations based on the child's condition, parents will have ultimate responsibility regarding the fate of their child. In certain situations where the parents are unavailable or negligent, that power may be removed by the court, and a guardian or guardian ad litem will be appointed to make those decisions instead.

Patients' Bill of Rights

The United States Patients' Bill of Rights was passed in 1998 to help strengthen consumer confidence in the health care system, and grant more patient autonomy in medical decisions. The U.S. Patients' Bill of Rights outlines eight major areas of health care decision-making. However, it's important to realize that these are just minimum standards, and each state has its own, sometimes more stringent, guidelines. The minimum standards include the following:

- **Information disclosure**. Patients have a right to receive information that is easily understandable regarding their health care plan, their health care provider, and their health care facility so that each patient has autonomy in making informed health care decisions.

- **Choice of providers and plans**. In order to ensure that each patient has access to high-quality health care, patients will have a choice of health care providers.

- **Access to emergency services**. Consumers have a right to access emergency medical services whenever and wherever the need arises; health plans should also provide payment for these services.

- **Participation in treatment decisions**. Patients have a right to be involved in their health care decisions. Those patients who are unable to participate for reasons of incompetence, or other reasons, have the right to be represented by a patient advocate—a parent, family member, guardian, or Guardian Ad Litem.

- **Respect and nondiscrimination**. Consumers must not be discriminated against in the delivery of health care services consistent with the benefits covered in their policy or as required by law. Consumers who are eligible for coverage under the terms and conditions of a health plan or program or as required by law must not be discriminated against in marketing and enrollment practices based on race, ethnicity, national origin, religion, sex, age, mental or physical disability, sexual orientation, genetic information, or source of payment.

- **Confidentiality of health information**. Patients have a right to confidentiality when it comes to their health care, and have a right to protection of their personal health information. Patients also have a right to their medical records. They are able to review them and receive copies of them.
- **Complaints and appeals**. All consumers have the right to a fair and efficient process for resolving differences with their health plans, health care providers, and health care facilities, including a system of internal review and an independent system of external review.
- **Consumer responsibilities**. Consumers are expected to play an active role in protecting their own health. Greater individual involvement by consumers in their care increases the likelihood of achieving the best outcomes, and helps support a quality improvement, cost-conscious environment. Ways in which parents can become involved include being active participants in all health care decisions, complying with treatment plans created by the provider, reading and understanding all documentation, and educating themselves about

health care benefits and coverage, including the appeals process.

Again, it's important to understand that the Patients' Bill of Rights differs from state to state, and in many cases they are more stringent than the minimum guidelines listed above. An overview of the regulations can be found at the United States Department of Health and Human Services, while individual state doctrines can be found through your state department.

Access to Medical Records

As the parent of the patient, you own the information contained within your child's medical records and have the right to request a copy of those records at any time. This goes back to one of the main tenets of the Patients' Bill of Rights: consumer responsibility. It is not only the provider's job to give the patient the necessary documentation, but it's also the parent of the patient's job to ask for it if it is not provided to them.

In order to obtain a copy of any medical records, the parent must request the copy in writing or fill out a medical release form. Many medical release forms refer to a privacy notice that the facility or provider must provide the patient. This privacy notice outlines what the provider can do with the patient's medical records and information, and how the patient can get access to their medical records.

The Health Insurance Portability and Accountability Act

The legal rules regarding who is allowed access to the child's medical records are detailed in the Health Insurance Portability and Accountability Act (HIPAA). While health care privacy has become somewhat synonymous with HIPAA, it is, in reality, only one part of what HIPAA covers. The Privacy Rule located in Title II specifically discusses Protected Health Information (PHI), which is defined as information about health status, provision of health care, or payment for health care. The guidelines set forth in the Privacy Rule include the same information as the privacy notification that the patient receives when visiting a provider or becoming a member of a health plan. A quick overview of the guidelines is listed below. Please note that "covered entity" refers to a health care provider that conducts certain transactions in electronic form, a health care clearinghouse, or a health plan.

1. A covered entity may disclose PHI to facilitate treatment, payment, or health care operations, or if the covered entity has obtained authorization from the individual.
2. A covered entity must make a reasonable effort to disclose only the minimum necessary information required to achieve its purpose. Covered entities must notify patients of how their PHI may be used.

3. A complaint process must be in place for each covered entity that a patient can access if there is a problem with the distribution of PHI.

4. Patients also have recourse outside of the covered entity. A patient can file an official complaint with the United States Department of Health and Human Services, Office for Civil Rights, if the patient feels the covered entity is not abiding by the Privacy Rule. Procedures have been established to investigate HIPAA violations, which can lead to payment of civil penalties.

Reasons to Sign a Third-Party Release

You, as the parent of the child, have the right to deny access of those records to certain third parties. It's your job to determine whether it makes sense to release the information to the requesting party, and to assess the potential benefits and ramifications of doing so.

There are many reasons why someone might want access to your child's medical records, but the two most common reasons are treatment and payment. When it comes to treatment, records are released to those involved in the child's care and treatment—doctors, specialists, and other medical professionals. When it comes to payment, the information is usually provided to the patient's insurance company.

Now, we know how you're feeling. At this point it's quite

likely that you feel overwhelmed by the amount of paperwork you've had to deal with. Many times parents are so concerned with the health and well-being of their child—and so overwhelmed—that when a request to release information come their way they sign it without knowing or caring what information the release pertains to.

But pay special attention here. If an insurance company asks you to sign paperwork giving them full access to your child's medical records, put down your pen immediately! It's always prudent to talk to your lawyer first to determine whether certain information should be released to your insurance company. As a general rule of thumb, always ask the insurance company what specific information they need, check with your lawyer to determine that it makes sense to release the information, and then request the information from the hospital or facility yourself. Once you have it in hand, you can forward it to the insurance company.

In some situations the parent may want to release the medical records to an interested party, such as a lawyer, primary care physician, or school. This will also require the parent to fill out a form or send a letter giving the hospital or medical professional permission. The hospital or medical facility that is treating your child is *not* allowed to release information to insurance companies or any other third party without a properly signed and dated authorization.

Is there any information that can be released without

parental consent? Information related to an injury that results from things like violence, child abuse, poisoning, or illegal activities *can* be released to the police and other governmental agencies without parental consent.

"Not Confidential" Information

In addition, the hospital may release information that's considered "not confidential" to the press and other sources. This includes information such as the child's name, address, age, and details of the accident. If you are the parent of a child who has been in an accident, and you don't want your child's information to become part of a front-page news story, you should tell the hospital you don't want this information released without your prior consent. Unless you give specific instructions not to release this information, this information may be released.

Family and Medical Leave Act

When a child has been seriously injured it's likely that one parent—and sometimes both parents—need to take a significant amount of time off from work to attend to more important matters. This means that in addition to worrying about the health and well-being of their child, parents also worry about keeping their jobs.

The Family and Medical Leave Act is federally mandated legislation designed to provide job protection in these types of situations. The Family and Medical Leave Act allows parents to take unpaid leave for a reasonable amount of time—up to 12 weeks—to care for a child with a "serious" health condition. "Serious" is defined as any physical or mental condition that requires inpatient hospital care or continual treatment.

However, the Family and Medical Leave Act does *not* apply to all people. In order to qualify, you must have worked at least 1,250 hours over a twelve-month period, for an employer that employs at least fifty people who have worked a twenty-hour workweek that year.

Those who qualify for the Family and Medical Leave Act are entitled to return to their previous position, or to a position that is equal in responsibility and payment, at the end of their leave. The same insurance benefits provided during the time the employee was working must also be honored during the time the employee is on leave.

There is only one situation in which reinstatement can be denied, and that is when the employee is among the top 10 percent in salary and reinstatement would cause economic hardship to the company. In this case the employee must receive notice that reinstatement is being denied. The employer is required by law to provide health insurance for up to twelve weeks. Here are some other things that are important to know about the Family and Medical Leave Act:

- The employee is required to request leave at least thirty days in advance.
- The employee must take all leave at once, unless other arrangements are approved by the employer.
- The employer can require that the employee use vacation time or other paid leave as part of the twelve weeks. For example, if you have two vacation weeks per year, and are requesting twelve weeks of leave, the employer only has to grant ten weeks of unpaid leave.

Required Certification

In many cases, employers will require certification by a health care provider before they grant leave. The certification will give the date and estimated duration of the condition, and will also state why the parent is needed.

While it doesn't happen that often, an employer can request a second opinion. If that second opinion differs from the first opinion, a third opinion is sought. It's important to note that all opinions after the first opinion must be paid for by the employer.

When an Employer Does Not Comply with the Act

A person who is terminated or not reinstated for taking leave can sue in either federal or state court, and is eligible for certain damages. An employee has up to two years to file suit, up to three if it's determined that the violation was willful. The Family and Medical Leave Act can be complex; if your request is denied, be sure to seek some help to determine whether the denial is legal.

PART III

Conditions and Treatments: What Does the Future Hold?

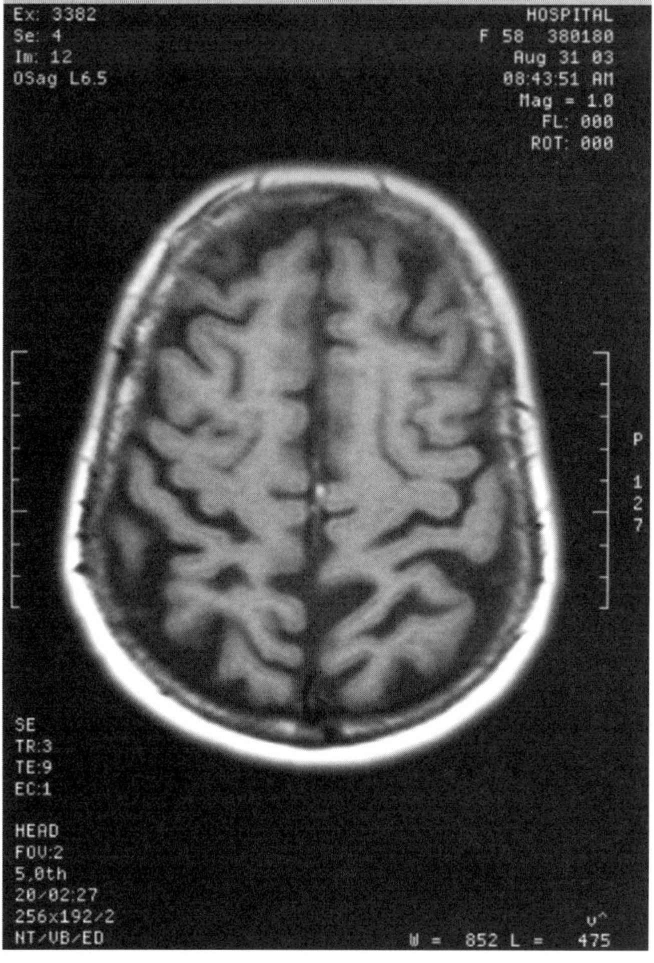

Some of your earliest concerns following your child's injury will be centered on your child's diagnosis and prognosis, and what that means in the near and long-term future. This section talks about specific conditions, as well as potential treatments.

Your Child's Diagnosis and Prognosis

Emergency room doctors are trained to—and required to—recognize serious medical conditions and treat them immediately. As soon as your child enters the emergency room she will be admitted and stabilized right away. This stabilization will attend to any life-threatening injuries, and will also ensure injuries don't get worse, or cause additional complications.

The process of diagnosing the brain injury begins almost immediately. It's important that the medical team knows right away if the child has experienced an injury, such as a depressed skull fracture, hematoma, or elevated intracranial pressure, because these types of injuries may require immediate surgery. If these injuries are not immediately diagnosed and the appropriate medical measures are not taken in a timely manner, your child's prognosis may end up much more dire than it needs to be.

Your child will be assessed for cognitive and physical impairment. He will most likely be asked a battery of questions and given some simple commands to determine how well he comprehends what's going on, as well as whether there are any issues with movement, speaking, or maintaining consciousness. Neurological signs, such as increased reflexes and muscle tone (which may be referred to by your child's doctor as "spasticity"), slurring of speech, difficulty swallowing or speaking, and tremors, may also indicate your child has sustained a moderate to severe brain injury.

Any child who has lost consciousness—even if it's for a short period of time—should undergo diagnostic tests that will allow the medical team to determine if bones of the skull have been fractured, and if any bone fragments have penetrated the skull and entered brain tissues. These tests will most likely include X-rays, CT scans, and MRI scans. Depending upon your child's specific circumstances, other tests might include an angiogram, ICP monitor, or electroencephalograph (EEG).

While it's difficult to predict the extent of recovery of a brain-injured patient, the type and extent of the injury, as well as the child's level of consciousness, can help the doctor make some loose predictions. To assess the level of consciousness, doctors use a tool called the Glasgow Coma Scale. This tool assesses the child's ability to move, speak, and open her eyes. As a general rule of thumb, the higher the score the better chance the child has of complete recovery. Scores of 8 or below are associated with severe brain injury, scores between 9 and 12 are associated with moderate brain injury, and scores above 13 indicate mild brain injury. In addition, the length of the coma is also used to determine the severity of the injury and the chances of recovery. For example, a child who has been unconscious for twenty minutes or less points toward a mild brain injury, while a child who has been in a coma for more than twenty minutes but for less than six hours indicates a moderate brain injury. A child who is in a coma for more than six hours has likely sustained a severe brain injury.

Glasgow Coma Scale

Eye Opening

4 = Responds spontaneously

3 = Responds to voice

2 = Responds to pain

1 = No response

Best Motor Response

6 = Follows commands

5 = Localizes to pain

4 = Withdraws to pain

3 = Decorticate (produces an exaggerated posture of upper extremity flexion and lower extremity extension in response to pain)

2 = Decerebrate (produces an exaggerated posture of extension in response to pain)

1 = No response

Best Verbal Response

5 = Oriented and converses

4 = Disoriented and converses

3 = Inappropriate words

2 = Incomprehensible sounds

1 = No sounds

It's important for parents to remember that brain injuries are extremely complex. Even "mild" brain injuries can have long-lasting effects that require your child to use coping skills for the rest of her life—problems that might be associated with memory, fatigue, emotions, and focus, among other things.

You need to accept that it may take years to completely understand the extent of your child's injuries. No two brain injuries behave exactly alike, making definitive outcomes impossible. For example, a brain injury that is diagnosed as "mild" may result in a long-term issue, or combination of long-term issues, that dramatically affect a child's life. On the other hand, some children who experience "severe" injuries recover to the point of leading lives that are similar to their lives before the injury.

Acquired Brain Injury

Jill was a happy, normal five-year-old until the SUV her grandfather was driving hit a patch of ice and rolled over three times. Now a teenager, Jill has made some recovery since the accident. However, she still suffers from severe cognitive impairment, physical issues, and wild mood swings. Jill is not able to care for herself, and requires constant supervision and support at school and at home.

Acquired brain injury is defined as any type of brain injury occurring after birth that is not caused by a congenital disorder or degenerative disease. There are two kinds of acquired brain injury: traumatic brain injury is the result of damage caused by an accident, such as a blow to the head or deceleration, while non-traumatic brain injury is caused by oxygen deprivation or by physical diseases or disorders such as stroke.

Common causes of acquired brain injury include automobile accidents, falls, sports-related injuries, automobile malfunctions, violence, choking, near-drowning, lead poisoning, and birth-related injuries.

Incidence of Acquired Brain Injury in Children

People between the ages of sixteen and twenty-five are at the highest risk for acquired brain injury. Preschoolers make up the second highest risk group. About one million children per year will sustain a head injury, and about 165,000 of those will require hospitalization. For every ten children who suffer from a brain injury, one of them will have a more serious injury that is classified as moderate or severe. Traumatic brain injury is the leading cause of death for children and young adults.

How Brain Injury in Children Differs from Brain Injury in Adults

First of all, all head injuries—whether suffered by an adult or a child—are classified as mild, moderate, or severe. The medical team will classify your child's head injury based on things such as the severity of the injury and how long a period of time, if any, your child experienced unconsciousness. Your child's brain injury will also be characterized as closed, meaning that the injury occurred to the skull only, or penetrating, meaning that the injury pierced brain tissues as well. A brain injury can be focal in nature, meaning it only affects one part of the brain, or it can be diffuse, affecting the entire brain. When it comes to symptoms and long-lasting effects, no two acquired brain injuries behave completely alike. Symptoms that occur initially following the accident might include headaches, altered consciousness, dizziness, blurred vision, personality changes, sleep disturbances, cognitive issues, and muscle problems. How long these symptoms last—whether they resolve themselves over time or are long-lasting and life-altering—will vary from child to child.

One thing that almost all parents want to know is whether there is a surefire way to predict how much of a recovery the child will make over time. Indeed, some of the symptoms that kids exhibit immediately following a head injury are quite sobering, and most parents want some assurance that there will be some improvement. At the very least, they want to know what to expect over the years.

However, head injuries that occur in children are particularly unpredictable, for the most part because the brains and central nervous systems of kids are still developing. Because of this, some features of brain injury are specific to kids. To explain what we mean, let's look at an example of a head injury in a typical adult. It's fairly easy to measure cognitive issues and personality changes in adults. For example, if Bob had a huge IQ and was an engineer prior to his accident, but after his accident no longer has the cognitive ability to do his job, you can be fairly certain that his head injury has caused cognitive impairment. If Sally was laid-back and easygoing prior to slipping and hitting her head, but is now anxious and short-tempered, it's fair to say that these personality changes are the result of her accident.

When it comes to kids, however, it's a lot tougher to measure the loss of brain function. Kids don't have job histories to draw on, their personalities aren't fully developed, and in some cases there are no records pertaining to IQ or academic performance. Some effects, of course, are very obvious. If the child has suffered from a severe brain injury that results in catastrophic injuries like loss of limb function or a major cognitive disability, the medical team can predict, to some degree, what the future holds. That being said, the full effects of brain injury may not be fully understood or realized for years. For example, the effects of frontal lobe injuries sustained by a very young child may not fully present themselves until the child is a teenager. That's because frontal lobe functions—functions such as interpersonal skills and social awareness—aren't fully developed until adolescence. And here's another example: it won't be possible to determine whether a child who isn't reading or writing at the time of the injury may have trouble in those areas as a result of the injury until he or she reaches school age.

Why is it important that all parents of brain-injured children realize that the effects of the injury can present themselves a long time—sometimes even years—down the road?

It is important that parents of all kids with brain injuries—whether those injuries are severe or mild—receive the support and services that are due to them. For example, even children with the mildest of head injuries are granted certain educational opportunities under federal law 94-142. Because no two brain injuries present themselves exactly alike, parents should have a lengthy discussion with their child's medical team that details exactly what kind of injury the child has sustained and what current symptoms and cognitive effects the child is experiencing, as well as any potential symptoms and cognitive effects the child may experience down the road. In addition to more immediate and obvious cognitive, emotional, and physical effects of brain injury, problems that may show up in the future include impaired executive function, lack of organizational skills, inappropriate behavior, social issues, ADD or ADHD, lack of motivation, an inability to problem solve, and irritability and opposition. Knowing exactly how the injury is affecting your child—or has the potential to affect your child—will ensure that you take full advantage of the support and services available to you.

Effects that Occur as a Result of Damage to Specific Areas of the Brain

Damage to the forehead area of the brain (frontal lobe) may result in:

- Paralysis
- Inability to express thoughts
- Inability to complete multi-step tasks
- Difficulty solving problems
- Issues with focus
- Social behavior changes
- Emotional and personality changes

Damage to the area near the back and top of head (parietal lobe) may result in:

- Trouble dealing with more than one object at a time
- Language difficulties, including remembering words in speech and in writing, and problems reading
- Difficulty with math
- Difficulty drawing
- Problems with spatial awareness

- Difficulty focusing the eyes
- Issues with hand-eye coordination
- Problems telling left from right

Damage to the back of the head (occipital lobes) may result in:

- Problems related to vision, including identifying colors, hallucinating, and difficulty locating objects
- Problems related to recognition, including the inability to recognize words, drawn objects, and the movement of an object
- Issues with reading and writing

Damage to the sides of the head above the ears (temporal lobes) might result in:

- Difficulty identifying and naming objects
- Short- and long-term memory loss
- Difficulty understanding spoken language
- Difficulty recognizing faces
- Sexual disturbances
- Excessive talking
- Aggressive behavior

Damage that occurs in the middle of the brain (brain stem) may result in:

- Difficulties perceiving the environment
- Difficulty breathing
- Difficulty with speech
- Difficulty swallowing
- Dizziness and nausea
- Issues with movement
- Issues with balance
- Sleep disturbances

Damage that occurs to the base of the skull (cerebellum) may result in:

- Inability to manage fine motor movement
- Inability to reach out for or grab objects
- Inability to walk
- Slurred speech
- Shaking or tremors
- Dizziness

Cost of Acquired Brain Injury

The cost of a brain injury varies according to which statistics you access. However, it is estimated that the cost of a severe injury is approximately $3 million, the cost of a moderate injury is approximately $941,000, and the cost of a mild injury is $85,000. Of course, it's impossible to put a price on the emotional and physical price both the child and his or her loved ones will pay as a result of the injury.

Three Stages of Treatment for Acquired Brain Injury

There are three stages of treatment for acquired brain injury.

Stage One: Acute Treatment

Chances are, by the time you are reading this your child has already gone through the acute treatment phase. This is the emergency treatment phase when all possible measures are taken to save your child's life and minimize the damage to the brain. Your child will be taken to the nearest hospital qualified to deal with brain injury cases, where stabilization and prevention of other medical conditions as a result of the accident will occur. If surgery is needed it will be done during this phase. In addition, the brain will be constantly monitored for swelling and pressure. Tests designed to determine the extent and location of the injury, such as the MRI and CT scans, may also be administered during this phase.

Many parents want to know how long their child will be in the hospital. The answer to that question depends upon the type and severity of the injury. As a general rule of thumb, children will remain in the intensive care unit (ICU) until any life-threatening injuries are stabilized. At that point, they'll be moved to a floor on the hospital that specializes in neurological issues such as brain injury. In many cases the child will then be transferred to a rehabilitation facility.

For now, we just want to let you know that at the same time you're coming to terms with your child's condition, you'll also be faced with some overwhelming medical discussions regarding the longer-term care of your child. Some of these conversations may seem to come at you quickly. Take a deep breath, and keep a cool head. Slow the conversations down if you don't like the pace at which they're going. When it comes to the health care options for your child beyond the ICU and neurological wing, ask lots of questions, then review the answers and ask more. There are lots of things that will factor into your decisions—your child's particular injuries, the location of the facility, and how much it costs and whether you can afford it. Be sure to take notes, and if you find your head is spinning, try recording your meetings.

How Do You Answer Your Child's Questions?

The days and weeks following your child's injury will be very difficult for him. As your child struggles with the cognitive and physical impairments that result from the injury, he's likely to go through a wide range of emotions including confusion, anger, denial, and fear. It's important that you help your child through this difficult time so he can focus on getting better. So how do you do that?

Your child will likely have lots of questions regarding the accident. Answer them as honestly as possible. The goal should be to tell the truth while still maintaining a positive, hope-filled attitude. It's important that your child understand, to the extent that his age and injury allows, what has happened and what the prognosis is. It may take your child a little while to accept what's happened, but acceptance is an important precursor to getting well. If your child doesn't accept what has happened, he can't take the steps necessary to recovery.

Sometime parents wonder how much help they should give their child, especially if their child is older and somewhat independent. While it may be intuitive to ease the mental and physical burdens on your child by doing everything you can for him, allowing your child to perform the tasks he is able to, while giving help when asked, is the best course of action.

Stage Two: Subacute Treatment

This phase begins after the patient is stabilized and continues until the patient either returns to the community or enters a long-term care facility. This phase usually takes place at a rehabilitation hospital, and is designed to help the child return to the maximum amount of function. During this time your child will work with a team of doctors, physical therapists, occupational therapists, speech therapists, and psychologists. Depending upon the extent of the injury, this phase can last for a couple of weeks to a year or even more. At the end of this phase, the child will be returned to either the home or to a long-term care facility.

Rehabilitation

Once your child has passed through the acute phase of care, he will begin the rehabilitation phase. The goal of this phase is to return your child to the maximum amount of function possible.

If your child's head injury is moderate to severe, there's a good chance that she will need to enter a rehabilitation center. In some cases the child will visit the rehabilitation center on an outpatient basis, but more often than not, your child will experience this phase as an inpatient of the hospital.

Choosing a Rehabilitation Facility for Your Child

Finding the right rehabilitation program for your child is extremely important for his future. The most important factor is whether or not the services and skills offered at the facility suit your child's specific needs. Other factors that frequently factor into a family's decision include proximity to the family home, and whether or not the facility is covered by the child's insurance.

The first order of business is to ensure that the facilities you are considering have the proper designation and accreditation. Facilities that have been recognized by the Commission on Accreditation of Rehabilitation Facilities (CARF) meet a certain standard of care, and generally offer a better variety of services. You can contact CARF by calling 1.520.325.1044, or by logging on to www.carf.org.

In addition, the Department of Health's Joint Commission on Accreditation of Healthcare Organizations (JCAHO) also designates certain facilities Brain and Spinal Cord Injury Program (BSCIP) facilities. In order to earn this designation, the facility must be accredited by CARF in brain injury, and must admit a certain amount of brain injury patients per year.

Finally, there are fourteen Model Systems Centers located throughout the United States. These facilities are considered the best in the nation. For more information on these centers, their locations, and what kinds of services they offer, check out www.msktc.washington.edu.

Once you have found facilities with the proper designation and accreditation, it's important to visit them to ensure that the program at the facility will suit your child. Below is a list of questions you should ask during your interview. This list of questions is by no means exhaustive, but rather serves as a jumping-off point.

1. Does the facility have experience treating children with brain injury?
2. What percentage of your patients are currently kids with brain injury?
3. Are there currently children of similar age and gender to mine being treated at the facility?
4. Do the kids in the brain injury program have similar injuries in terms of type and severity?
5. How many children with brain injuries were admitted in the last year?
6. Is the staff well trained in the specific needs of kids with brain injury?
7. Will my child's rehabilitation program include both short-term and long-term goals?
8. What kinds of specialists are on staff at the facility?

9. Is there anyone at the facility who will help us navigate insurance issues and other financial matters?

10. Is there physician coverage 24 hours a day, seven days a week?

11. How often will my child receive treatment? Will he or she receive treatment at least three hours per day?

12. What kinds of recreation and entertainment is available for my child?

13. How will we, as parents, be included in the rehabilitation process?

14. Will my child and other family members receive counseling as part of the treatment process?

Stage Three: Chronic Treatment

Many acquired brain injuries have long-term effects that require intervention over the course of the child's lifetime. These long-term effects generally vary in severity. Less severe long-term effects can be handled in the community, while more severe long-term effects may require that the child be treated in a chronic care facility. Children who can be treated in their community may opt for individual therapy at home, or they may attend an outpatient clinic on a regular basis. Children with more complex physical, medical, and social programs may benefit from a case-managed program, in which a case manager comes up with a course of action using the services of a team of physical therapists, occupational therapists, speech therapists, and psychologists.

One area that is sometimes overlooked but that is incredibly important to the gains a child makes following an injury is social support. At some point during the treatment phase the child will reach a point where he no longer seems to be making any gains. When this happens, it's important that the medical team, as well as family and friends, band together to give the child the support he needs.

In some cases, the injuries that result from the acquired brain injury will be so profound that the child will not be able to be cared for at home. In situations where the child requires skilled nursing care, a long-term care facility that specializes in brain-injured children is the best option.

Cerebral Palsy

Nathan's mother enjoyed a normal pregnancy, but endured a difficult labor. After many hours of unproductive labor things still weren't moving along. The doctor attempted to deliver the child with forceps and a vacuum, but the child still was not descending properly. At this time monitors showed a significant decrease in Nathan's heart rate—enough of a decrease to cause lack of oxygen to the brain. Today Nathan is a five-year-old child with cerebral palsy. Nathan is confined to a wheelchair, and has problems with his vision and hearing. Nathan attends a mainstream classroom with the help of a full-time aid and an independent educational plan (IEP) that has been designed with his specific learning disabilities in mind.

Cerebral palsy (CP) is a medical condition that results from permanent brain injury to one of the motor control centers to the brain, or to one of the pathways to these centers. Because the disorder affects the movement center of the brain, the primary symptom of cerebral palsy is a lack of muscle movement and control. Depending upon exactly which areas of the brain have been affected, the child might experience muscle spasms, involuntary movement, mobility issues, and problems with gait. However, along with movement disorders, CP is also commonly associated with mental retardation, blindness, loss of hearing, spasms, learning disorders, and seizures. Most cases of cerebral palsy are identified immediately after birth, though it's not unheard of for a diagnosis to be made later in childhood.

If you are like lots of parents, you probably want to know *why* your child has cerebral palsy. Quite simply, your child has cerebral palsy because her brain has been damaged. Of course, if you are like most parents you are now going to ask the logical follow-up question. Why does my child have brain damage?

That question is a little tougher because it's not always possible to know for sure what caused the brain damage that resulted in cerebral palsy. We do know that cerebral palsy is caused by an injury to the brain before, during, or shortly after birth, but it's not always possible to say when the injury occurred, or what caused it. Some cases are thought to be the result of a developmental brain formation during pregnancy, while other cases are thought to be the result of neurological damage during or shortly after birth.

About 10 to 15 percent of cases of cerebral palsy can be attributed to a recognized brain injury such as bleeding into the brain, an infection, or damage caused by lack of oxygen. Some of these situations are preventable, and are the result of mistakes made during the birth process. That being said it's not possible for the typical parent to determine whether their child's cerebral palsy was the result of a preventable mistake. Rather, this is a complex determination that requires careful study by a qualified medical and legal team. Preventable causes of brain injury that cause cerebral palsy include the following:

- Central nervous system infections and streptococcal infections in the mother during pregnancy
- Birth trauma, specifically trauma that causes lack of oxygen caused by an interruption of breathing during or around the time of birth

- Neonatal jaundice
- Central nervous system traumas, such as near drowning
- Infections during early childhood, such as meningitis

Prognosis of Cerebral Palsy

One of the first things that parents want to know is whether there is a "cure" for cerebral palsy. While CP isn't a progressive disorder—in other words, it doesn't get worse over time—there is no cure. Cerebral palsy is a permanent condition that will likely affect how your child lives and plays for the rest of her life. While this may seem like a grim statement, parents can rest assured that there are plenty of treatment options specifically designed to increase the quality of life for children with CP.

Cost of Cerebral Palsy

Cerebral palsy is the second most expensive developmental disability to manage, with estimated costs of $1 million over the course of an individual's lifetime.

Traditional Treatment Options for Brain Injury and CP

These treatments are more likely to be covered by insurance and government benefit programs. To ensure maximum benefits, these treatments should be initiated as soon as possible because early intervention has been shown to have a significant positive impact on kids with CP.

Special note to parents of children with CP: While we mentioned earlier that CP is not progressive, the symptoms can worsen over time if muscles and bones aren't used. Frequently, patients who don't receive adequate therapy develop arthritis. Most effective treatments for CP are long term, and should be implemented consistently, over the course of the child's life.

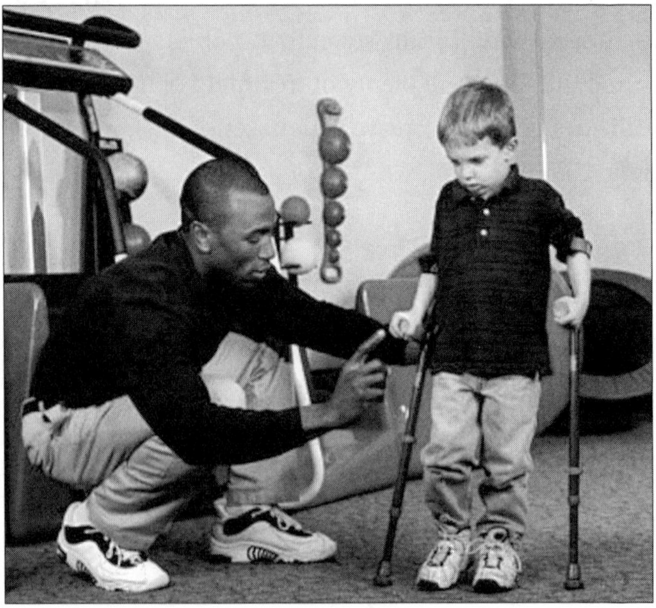

Physical Therapy

Some children with brain injuries develop issues with movement and muscles, and physical therapy is needed to return them to a maximum amount of function. Physical therapy is probably the single most important therapy for a child with CP because it promotes the proper use of muscles and increases muscle strength. Physical therapy needs to be used throughout the life of the CP patient. The amount of physical therapy needed for children with CP varies from person to person.

Speech Therapy

Some special needs children need to relearn how to speak, specifically how to use the muscles in their faces and mouths. Even though physical therapy focuses on the use of muscles, it often neglects the use of facial muscles that are important in communication, eating, and breathing. Speech therapy focuses on the use and strengthening of the facial muscles, along with other muscles found in the jaw and head.

Occupational Therapy

This therapy focuses on tasks and movements that will allow your child to be more independent. Instead of being body focused like physical therapy, occupational therapy tends to be more task-oriented, with body movement becoming a consequential act of the task. This type of therapy will allow the child to participate in everyday activities such as feeding, dressing, and bathing. Children with brain injury require occupational therapy to get them to maximum function, while children with CP often require occupational therapy over the course of their entire lives.

Massage Therapy

This therapy is important to the overall health of your child because it assists in decreasing the tenseness often associated with CP, and increases joint flexibility. Massage can be integral in helping your child have more control over his or her body.

Counseling

Counseling is an important part of the overall treatment plan because many kids with special needs are faced with emotional disturbances that are caused by their physical condition. Counseling should always be part of a complete treatment plan for anyone suffering from a disability, especially if it is a long-term or lifelong disability.

Recreational Therapy

Recreational therapy shows kids with special needs that it's possible to play and have fun. Treatment often includes showing kids how to adapt to certain hobbies and sports, taking their limitations into consideration.

The Use of Complementary and Alternative Medicine (CAM)

Complementary and alternative medicine (CAM) are therapies that are considered "unconventional." Even though most of these therapies have been around longer than "conventional" Western medicine, they are not widely accepted in the medical community due to lack of research. However, with increased funding from the National Institute of Health (NIH) and many private entities, CAM therapies are proving to be beneficial in many diseases and illnesses that Western medicine has failed to treat or control. CAM therapies appear to be especially effective in patients with chronic conditions, such as diabetes, chronic back and neck pain, osteoarthritis, and gastrointestinal conditions. Many people with disabilities suffer from chronic conditions, especially pain, joint stiffness, constipation, and skin infections. All CAM therapies are an excellent complement to their conventional treatment plan. Users of CAM therapies have noted that use of CAM decreases their need for conventional medicine, subsequently lowering their bills as the need for medications and doctor's visits decrease. Additionally, CAM offers a more holistic approach to medicine, compared to conventional Western medicine, and users of CAM report an increased sense of well-being. CAM users also tend to have more control over their health care decisions, which can also ultimately lead to increased overall health. Many CAM therapies are proving to be beneficial for children with special needs to help them manage their symptoms and improve their quality of life.

Common CAM modalities include the following:

Acupuncture

Acupuncture, one of the major traditional Chinese medicines, originated in China more than 2,000 years ago and has been used in the United States since the early 1970s. The most common acupuncture technique involves the insertion of thin, metallic needles into the skin at a very superficial level, and the needles are then either manually manipulated or electrically stimulated, depending on the type of treatment. Due to standardizations of training on a state level, many health insurance companies now pay for acupuncture treatments. Some insurance companies require preauthorization for acupuncture treatments.

Osteopathic and Chiropractic Therapies

Osteopathic and chiropractic therapies fall under the blanket term of "manipulative medicine." Chiropractic medicine focuses more on the musculoskeletal and nervous systems of the body and how these systems are affected in a disease process, while osteopathic medicine also focuses on the musculoskeletal and nervous systems. Almost all insurance policies will pay for manipulative treatment from a chiropractor or osteopath. However, some policies have limitations as to how many times a year one can get manipulative therapies.

Reiki

Reiki is a form of energy medicine and is based on the theory that changes in energy within the body are the cause of disease and illness. Reiki practitioners are trained to detect these changes and bring the flow of energy within the body back to normal. Most insurance companies will not pay for Reiki therapy.

Massage Therapy

In addition to acupuncture and manipulative therapies, massage therapy is one of the most highly regulated and perhaps most researched CAM therapies. Massage therapy differs from manipulative therapies in that it focuses on manipulation of only the muscles and soft tissues. If a physician prescribes massage therapy as part of a treatment plan, many insurance companies will pay for it.

Hyperbaric Oxygen Therapy

Hyperbaric oxygen therapy (HBOT) has been credited with decreasing many of the symptoms of CP. During HBOT, your child will be placed in a sealed pressure chamber, and will breathe 100 percent oxygen at a pressure below that of sea level. Each treatment lasts for about sixty to ninety minutes, and occurs five or six days a week over the course of the treatment. Most initial treatments comprise forty HBOT sessions, with a reevaluation by the medical team occurring after the initial phase of treatment.

How does being placed in a hyperbaric chamber help a child with cerebral palsy? Well, cerebral palsy is the result of a brain injury to a specific area of the brain. However, the decrease in blood flow—and subsequently oxygen—to the injured part of the brain may greatly affect the parts of the brain surrounding the damaged area. The cells in this larger area don't die, but the small amount of oxygen they are receiving causes them to "go to sleep." In addition, myelin sheaths—the coverings that protect the nerve fibers in the brain—may fail to develop. These nerve fibers play a key role in transmitting signals from the brain to the spinal cord, but when

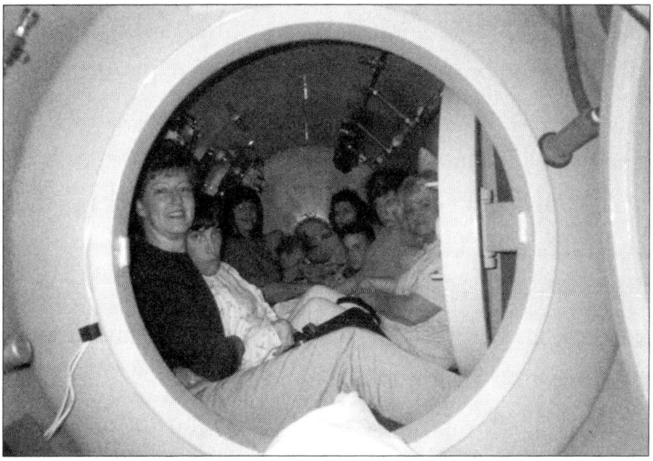

they aren't protected by myelin they eventually deteriorate. Communication between the brain and muscles breaks down, and the result may be spasticity.

However, when the "sleeping" cells are exposed to high levels of oxygen they "wake up," which allows the nerve cells to recover. The extra oxygen also contributes to the reduction of swelling in the brain, which allows new brain tissue to develop. The effects of HBOT can't be undermined—they are real, and they are documented. Recent studies, including one done in Quebec, Canada, and reported in Britain's most renowned medical journal, *The Lancet*, have concluded that HBOT may significantly assist a child with cerebral palsy. Like all CP therapies, early treatment is key. Most insurance companies routinely deny HBOT, but with strong advocacy and well-researched arguments they can be convinced to allow this benefit.

Hippotherapy

Hippotherapy comprises a combination of physical therapy and occupational therapy using horseback riding. The theory is that the movement of the horse allows the child's hips and core to move in the proper way, while also increasing balance and rhythm. Hippotherapy can help with muscle tone, coordination, mobility, posture, balance, and limbic system function, which in turn can improve gross motor skills such as sitting, standing, and walking. Hippotherapy has also been shown to contribute to the psychological and emotional well-being of kids with special needs. Few insurance policies cover Hippotherapy without convincing argument and advocacy.

Suit Therapy

This therapy is specifically designed for children with cerebral palsy, to help them achieve reduced spasticity, better muscle tone, and increased coordination. The suit the child wears is similar to those suits worn by Russian astronauts in the 1970s to prevent muscle atrophy. You can find suits specifically designed for CP therapy under the brand names TheraSuit, Adeli Suit, NeuroSuit, and Penguin suit.

The suit comprises four different pieces—a vest, shorts, kneepads, and shoes—that are attached with flexible cords. The cords can be adjusted based on the amount of tension on the child's muscles that is desired.

In a nutshell, the system allows the child to engage in resistance training, much like a weight workout at the gym. Suit therapy can be expensive, but could be one of the most effective treatments for kids with CP. If a suit therapy is part of your child's physical therapy experience your insurance company might pay for it. Getting your insurance company to pay for the use of the suit at home can be more difficult.

Aquatherapy

Aquatherapy, in which the child receives therapy in the water, is easier on the joints and bones, and allows children to exercise and move more freely. This kind of therapy can be very effective for special needs children who have muscle, movement, and coordination issues.

In addition to improving coordination and muscle tone, aquatherapy also allows kids, who otherwise might be unable, to improve their cardiovascular health through aerobic exercise.

Aquatherapy is usually covered under physical therapy in most insurance policies.

Botox Therapy

Botox injections, used in conjunction with physical therapy, can increase muscle relaxation, reduce spasticity, and increase the range of motion in children with

CP. Botox therapy is not approved by the FDA for treating CP, which means that in most cases insurance will not cover the treatment.

Who Pays for CAM?

Depending upon the specifics of an insurance policy, complementary and alternative medicines may be reimbursed anywhere from 50 to 100 percent. But as I noted above, many CAM therapies are not covered by insurance. Therapies such as massage therapy, osteopathic manipulative therapy, and chiropractic care, which have been more researched and more widely used and accepted in the United States, tend to have higher reimbursement rates than newer or lesser-known therapies. Many insurance companies decide on reimbursement based on research that has been done on the therapy. Little research will almost guarantee that the therapy will not be covered under the insurance plan. However, it is always prudent to contact the insurance company to determine which therapies will be covered. Also, it is important to keep in mind that even if some insurance companies cover a therapy, they may have limitations as to how many treatment sessions per year a patient can be reimbursed for. For example, even if an insurance company covers chiropractic care at 100 percent, this may be limited to ten visits per year, which means the eleventh visit will be paid by the patient at 100 percent out-of-pocket. Sometimes, if a physician prescribes the therapy, the insurance company will pay for it, but normally the reimbursement is not as high as it is with conventional therapies. If a patient is a frequent user of CAM therapies, it may be wise for that patient to seek out an insurance policy that is CAM-friendly.

PART IV

Education

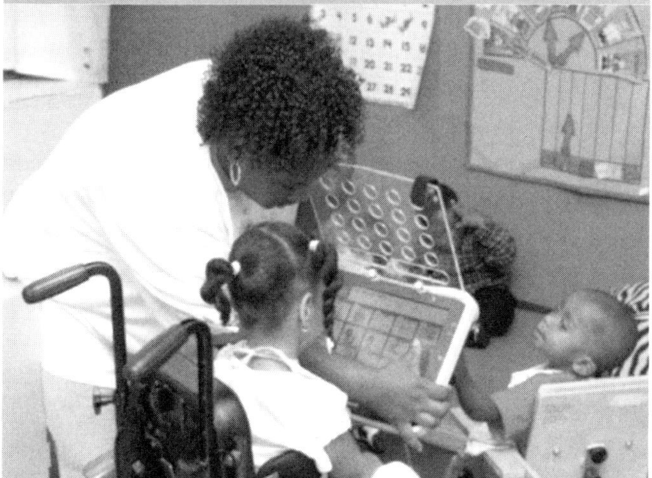

Upon being discharged from the rehabilitation facility, your child may require additional services at home. Depending upon the severity of your child's injury, these services will vary from inpatient rehabilitation to in-home nursing care.

However, when all is said and done, school ends up being the biggest provider of services to kids with special needs. That's because in 1990, as part of the Americans with Disabilities Act, the Individuals with Disabilities Education Act (IDEA) expanded to include brain injury as a disability category for children requiring special education services. One of your jobs as a parent is to ensure that your child receives the education that she deserves.

While the information below pertains mostly to children of school age, parents should know that in many cases, early intervention programs are available for any child who has physical or mental issues that will delay their progress in school. A toddler with CP or a brain injury can receive services from the school district well before that child reaches school age, if they meet certain qualifications. Be sure to talk to your school district to determine what kinds of early intervention programs are available for your child.

What Is IDEA?

The Individuals with Disabilities Education Act is a federal law that develops minimum guidelines regarding special education for children with disabilities from the time of birth to twenty-one years of age. IDEA was originally called the Education for All Handicapped Children Act (EHA), which was passed back in 1975. EHA was renamed IDEA in 1990, with major amendments in 1997 and 2004. This federal law provides federal funding to state and public agencies, and therefore governs how their programs administer early intervention and special education programs for disabled children. Every state is required to follow the rules and regulations of the IDEA. Part C of IDEA covers children from birth through two years of age, while Part B covers children from three years to twenty-one years of age.

Eligibility Requirements Under IDEA

Not every child with a disability will fall under IDEA, as the disability must have an adverse effect on the child's educational performance and his ability to progress in academics. There are specific requirements for defining a child with a disability, and it is defined under the Act as "a child with mental retardation, hearing impairments (including deafness), speech or language impairments, visual impairments (including blindness), serious emotional disturbance, orthopedic impairments, autism, traumatic brain injury, other health impairments, or specific learning disabilities; and who, by reason thereof, needs special education and related services." Children who do not fall under this definition may qualify for services under Section 504 of the Rehabilitation Act of 1973, or under the Developmental Disabilities Bill of Rights Act, or under the Americans with Disabilities Act.

Individualized Education Program

One of the most important provisions of IDEA is the individualized education program (IEP), which is a plan that is designed to meet the unique learning needs of each disabled child. If a child qualifies under state and federal disability guidelines, IDEA requires that each public school create an IEP for each eligible child. For each child, an IEP team is created to develop an IEP plan. The IEP team must include at least one of the child's parents and the parents are seen as equal members of the IEP team. Other members of the team include the child's teachers, school psychologists, and administrators, and the IEP must be developed jointly by school officials and the parents. The general requirements of the contents of an IEP include the following:

- A statement of the child's present levels of academic achievement and functional performance
- A statement of measurable annual goals, including academic and functional goals designed to do the following:
    - Meet the child's needs that result from the child's disability to enable the child to be involved in and make progress in the general education curriculum; and
    - Meet each of the child's other educational needs that result from the child's disability;
- How the child's progress toward meeting the annual goals are to be measured and reported to the parent
- A statement of the special education and related services and supplementary aids
- Schedule of services to be provided, including when the services are to begin and the frequency, duration, and location for the provision of services
- A statement of any individual appropriate accommodations that are necessary to measure the academic achievement and functional performance of the child on state- and district-wide assessments.

Additionally, if classroom accommodations are needed, these must be identified in the IEP and provided for by the public school system. If parents do not agree with the IEP, they are able to initiate the appeal process to voice their concerns. One of the goals of the IEP is to provide each child with a free appropriate public education (FAPE).

Free Appropriate Public Education

In 2004, IDEA was amended to include the right of a free appropriate public education (FAPE). FAPE is defined as special education and related services that have been provided at public expense, under public supervision and direction, and without charge; that meet the standards of the state educational agency; include an appropriate preschool, elementary school, or secondary school education in the state involved; and are provided in conformity with the child's individualized education program (IEP). The purpose of a FAPE is to provide the child with an education that prepares the child for further education, employment, and independent living.

Related Services

Section 602 of IDEA defines "related services" as services that a disabled child may be entitled to if these services assist the child with his or her educational needs.

Related services include:

- Transportation
- Speech-language pathology
- Audiology services
- Interpreting services
- Psychological services
- Physical and occupational therapy
- Recreation, including therapeutic recreation
- Social work services
- School nurse services designed to enable a child with a disability to receive a free appropriate public education as described in the individualized education program of the child
- Counseling services, including rehabilitation counseling
- Orientation and mobility services
- Medical services (except that such medical services shall be for diagnostic and evaluation purposes only) as may be required to assist a child with a disability to benefit from special education, and includes the early identification and assessment of disabling conditions in children.

It is a good idea to look into which of the services should be provided by the public school system for a disabled child and incorporate these services in the IEP.

The Rehabilitation Act of 1973

Section 504 of the Rehabilitation Act of 1973 outlines specific rights that are guaranteed to people with disabilities. When a disabled child does not qualify for assistance under IDEA because their disability does not fall under the IDEA definition, lawyers may oftentimes look under Section 504 to seek available resources. Section 504 states that no person with a disability will be excluded from participation in, be denied benefits of, or be subjected to discrimination under any program or activity receiving federal financial assistance. If a child qualifies under Section 504, then a 504 Plan may be created, which is similar to an IEP, but instead falls under the guidelines of the Rehabilitation Act.

PART V
Estate Planning

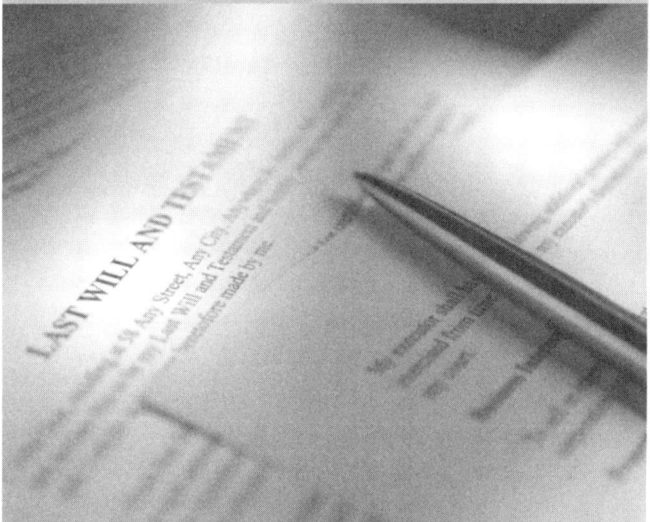

Parents of children with special needs face some very unique challenges when it comes to planning for their child's future medical and financial needs. While no parent likes to think of the tragic situations that might leave their child without him, it's important to have some peace of mind when it comes to how your child will be taken care of. Especially in cases where cognitive ability is impaired, it's important to know that steps are taken to manage your child's finances and care in the future.

Many parents don't bother with estate planning because they don't think they have enough assets. In most cases this isn't true. Some of the assets we hold—such as life insurance—aren't important in life but become very important in death. No matter how little you think you have, estate planning is necessary.

One of the factors that parents of special needs children must consider is whether their child will receive—or will one day receive—SSI, Medicaid, or other governmental benefits. Inheriting too many assets through your estate may render your child ineligible for these programs. Your lawyer can help you structure a special estate plan that will minimize impact on your child's long-range needs.

Guardianship

The laws regarding guardianship vary from state to state. In Pennsylvania, a guardian is a person who is legally allowed to make decisions that affect an incapacitated person's life. A guardian manages the incapacitated person's personal, legal, and financial affairs.

When the incapacitated person is an adult, the guardian is appointed by the court, and is usually a husband, wife, parent, or close relative that is deemed to have the incapacitated person's best interests at heart. In order to be named a guardian, a petition must be filed and a hearing must occur.

However, when the injured person is a child under the age of eighteen, the rules are completely different. Because parents are the natural guardians of their children, no petition needs to be filed.

What happens if the child reaches the age of eighteen and is still not able to make personal, financial, or legal decisions affecting his or her life? At that point, the parents will have to file a petition seeking guardianship. During the hearing, the judge will look at medical documentation to determine whether the individual is able to manage his or her own finances, health, and safety. If the judge determines the individual can't manage these things, a guardian will be appointed.

Parents should also name an "alternate guardian" in their will, should something happen to them. This alternate guardian will be responsible for making all the same decisions a parent would make.

Parents who suspect that their child's disabilities will require guardianship past the age of eighteen should meet with an attorney to make arrangements to ensure that their child's welfare will always be taken care of. It's difficult to imagine your child not being able to make decisions for himself or herself as an adult. It's difficult to imagine that you may not always be around to ensure that your child's best interests are taken care of. And these things are even more difficult to talk about. But in order to ensure that your child's needs are always met, the issue of guardianship must be discussed immediately with family members and your attorney.

An important reminder: because laws regarding guardianship vary from state to state, be sure you understand those that pertain to you.

Guardian Ad Litem

A guardian ad litem is an individual, usually an attorney, who is appointed by the court to ensure that the best interests of the child are met.

In situations where a child sustains a serious brain injury, a guardian ad litem may be appointed if both parents are deceased, or if they are unavailable for some reason. Another situation in which a guardian ad litem might be appointed is if the child lives with one parent, and that parent's negligence caused the accident that resulted in the brain injury. A petition must be filed in order for a guardian ad litem to be named, and is usually done so by a family member, a child welfare department, or an attorney.

The guardian ad litem is responsible for reviewing all legal and medical records, and meets with attorneys and doctors to determine what is in the best interest of the child. The guardian ad litem will ensure that proper legal actions are taken to ensure the child's rights, and is responsible for navigating things such as health care benefits, government benefits, and educational benefits, among other things.

Parents can avoid the possibility of a court-appointed guardian ad litem with careful estate planning. No parent wants to imagine not being there for their child, especially when their child has special needs. While the guardian ad litem system is designed to ensure that the child always has an advocate in their corner, most parents rest easier knowing that the person acting in their child's best interest is someone they know and trust.

Writing a Will

If you do not have a will at the time of your death, your assets will be distributed according to the laws of the state in which you live. Since distributing your assets without a will can take a long time and definitely isn't usually the best way to pass property on—especially when special circumstances should be taken into consideration—it's best to have a will.

While there are many "will kits" and websites that allow you to draw up your own will, the fact is that drawing up an effective will that gels with your circumstances is the kind of complicated task that requires the services of an experienced lawyer. In particular, seek out the services of a lawyer who has drafted wills for parents of children with disabilities.

Estate Planning Considerations

The first thing you should do is assess your child's disability, and determine what that means for your child's future. Will your child be able to make a living, or manage a household? Will she be able to handle her own finances? If your child is particularly young and it's hard to say what the future holds, err on the side of caution. You can always amend your estate plan as your child grows. You'll also need to consider whether or not your child will be able to live on her own in the event of your death. If your child is of the age that she requires care, or if your child's particular needs indicate that lifelong supervision is necessary, you'll have to recommend a guardian or conservator in your will.

Be sure to consider what kind of government benefits

your child is eligible to receive. Some benefits, such as SSDI, will remain unaffected by any assets your child inherits. Others, such as SSI and Medicaid, have financial eligibility requirements. Another category of government benefits charges for services based on the individual's ability to pay.

Next, take a careful look at your own finances. What is the worth of your estate should you die in the near future? Your attorney will help you craft your estate plan so that it remains somewhat flexible, in case your situation changes somewhat between the time you write your estate plan and your death.

Disinheriting Your Child

Parents of all children, whether they are disabled or not, have the right to disinherit their child. This means that no assets from your estate are left to your disinherited child.

In some cases, it makes sense to disinherit your special needs child, especially if you have modest assets and your child has costly needs. Disinheriting your child in this type of circumstance would allow your child to receive care through state and federal support after your death.

Gifts

Parents of a special needs child can leave that child an outright gift designed to take care of future needs, as long as that child is not receiving—or expected to receive in the future—government benefits. Outright gifts should only be left to brain-injured children who have no cognitive impairments, as they will need to make their own decisions when it comes to managing the gift.

Morally Obligated Gifts

A morally obligated gift is one you leave to your other child or children, with the stipulation that they will use the money to care for their disabled sibling. Morally obligated gifts are best when there are few assets to distribute and the disabled child does not require lifelong care or medical services. It's important to note that the child who is left the morally obligated gift is not required to spend it in the way the parent suggests.

Special Needs Trust

Setting up a special needs trust is one way to ensure that your child inherits assets but also gets to keep the government benefits that he needs.

People who receive government benefits often find themselves in somewhat of a financial bind. While the services they receive—for example, Medicaid—might be of considerable size, the amount of money they receive for normal living expenses is not enough to lift them above poverty level. Parents and charitable organizations may assist the brain-injured individual to improve his or her quality of life, but they must do so in a way that follows government regulations.

One of the best ways of doing this is through the special needs trust. A special needs trust supplements the child's resources in a way that doesn't interfere with her ability to receive government benefits. How does a special needs trust work? In a nutshell, the parent puts a certain amount of resources in the trust. A trustee is then responsible for disseminating funds as appropriate, on behalf of the child. This allows families to circumvent the rule that states that a person with a disability can't have a trust, as technically the trust does not belong to the person with the disability, but to the trustee. The trustee is given sole discretion when it comes to how funds are allocated.

While I've made it sound simple, the fact is that the rules and regulations surrounding special needs trusts are actually quite complicated—and stringent. To that end, it's imperative that anyone setting up a special needs trust for their child retain the services of an attorney who is very familiar not only with special needs trusts, but also how they might affect government benefit programs.

Intervivos Trust

An intervivos special needs trust, sometimes also called a living special needs trust, is a trust that functions while the parents are still living, and is designed to look after the future of the special needs child. An intervivos trust, which is set up as a checking account at a bank, can be established before a child turns eighteen. This trust allows parents to add money to be used in the future as well as to cover current supplementary expenses. This kind of trust is managed by the trustees (usually the parents), is kept separate from the family's main estate, and the expenses that come out of it are tax-deductible.

Because the parents of the child contribute money to the trust each month, and because they may have also transferred assets or life insurance to the trust, this kind of trust creates a very secure future for the brain-injured child should the parents pass away. The parents name a "successor trustee," who would take over the management of the fund for the disabled child if the parents were no longer able to. This allows the trust to function without interruption, ensuring that the child continues to get the care that she needs and requires.

Letter of Intent

A letter of intent is a document written by the parents or guardians that describes the brain-injured child's condition, his history, specific needs, and their wishes, hopes, and desires for their child's future. While not specifically a legal document, a letter of intent can guide the court and others involved in the future upbringing of your child. In addition, a letter of intent is a nice thing for your lawyer to have because she can ensure that all legal documents pertaining to your child are complimentary to your wishes. A letter of intent should be written right away, and should be updated frequently as your child's needs change. Areas to consider when writing a letter of intent include behavior management, education, employment, housing, medical history, religion, and social environment.

Disclaimer: *This book is not a substitute for professional advice, and does not constitute legal advice or an attorney/client relationship. The information in this book is general, and does not cover the laws of all states. For more information on state-specific laws, as well as legal answers that pertain to your specific circumstances, please seek the services of a qualified and experienced attorney.*

RESOURCES

General Resources

MUMS: National Parent to Parent Organization
Julie Gordon
150 Custer Court
Green Bay, WI 54301
Phone: 920.336.5333; Toll-free: 877.336.5333
E-mail: mums@netnet.net
Website: www.netnet.net/mums

Danielle's Foundation
"A non-profit resource for families of children with cerebral palsy & brain injuries"
One Liberty Place
1650 Market Street
Philadelphia, PA 19103
Toll free: 800.511.2283
E-mail: info@daniellesfoundation.org
Website: www.daniellesfoundation.org

Brain Injury Association of America
1608 Spring Hill Rd., Suite 110
Vienna, VA 22182
Phone: 703.761.0750
E-mail: info@biausa.org
Website: www.biausa.org

Brain Injury Resource Center

P.O. Box 84151
Seattle, WA 98124-5451
Phone: 206.621.8558
E-mail: brain@headinjury.com
Website: www.headinjury.com

National Association of Children's Hospitals and Related Institutions

401 Wythe Street
Alexandria, VA
Phone: 703.684.1355
E-mail: webmaster@nachri.org
Website: www.childrenshospitals.net

National Dissemination Center for Children with Disabilities

P.O. Box 1492
Washington, D.C. 20013
Phone: 202.884.8200; Toll-free: 800.695.0285
E-mail: nichcy@aed.org
Website: www.nichcy.org

United Cerebral Palsy

1660 L Street, NW
Suite 700
Washington, D.C. 20036
E-mail: info@ucp.org
Website: www.ucp.org

Education/Rehabilitation Resources

The American Occupational Therapy Association

4720 Montgomery Lane

Bethesda, MD 20824

Phone: 301.652.2682

Website: www.aota.org

American Physical Therapy Association

1111 North Fairfax Street

Alexandria, VA 22314

Phone: 800.999.2782

Website: www.apta.org

The American Therapeutic Recreation Association

1414 Prince St.

Suite 204

Alexandria, VA 22314

Phone: 703.683.9420

Website: www.atra-tr.org

Commission on Accreditation of Rehabilitation Facilities (CARF)

4891 E. Grant Rd.

Tucson, TX 85712

Phone: 520.325.1044; Toll-free 888.281.6531

Website: www.carf.org

E-mail: medical@carf.org

National Rehabilitation Information Center (NARIC)
8201 Corporate Drive, Suite 600
Landover, MD 20785
Phone: 301.459.5900; Toll-free 800.346.2742; TTY 301.459.5984
E-mail: info@naric.com
Website: www.naric.com

US Office of Special Education and Rehabilitation
US Department of Education
400 Maryland Avenue, SW
Washington, D.C. 20202
Phone: 800.872.5327
Website: www.ed.gov

Government Benefit Resources

Social Security Administration
Windsor Park Building
6401 Security Boulevard
Baltimore, MD 21235
Phone: 800.772.1213
Website: www.ssa.gov/disability

The National Organization of Social Security Claimants' Representatives
560 Sylvan Avenue
Englewood Cliffs, NJ 07632
Phone: 800.431.2804
Website: www.nosscr.org

Medicaid

Phone: 877.267.2323

Website: www.cms.hhs.gov/medicaid

Medicare

Phone: 800.MEDICARE

Website: www.medicare.gov

The Medicare Rights Center

1460 Broadway, 17th Floor

New York, New York 10036

Phone: 212.869.3850

Website: www.medicarerights.org

The Center for Medicare Advocacy

1101 Vermont Avenue, NW

Washington, D.C. 20005

Phone: 202.216.0028

Website: www.medicareadvocacy.org

National Institute on Disability and Rehabilitation Research, Office of Special Education and Rehabilitative Services, US Department of Education

U.S. Department of Education

400 Maryland Avenue, SW

Washington, D.C. 20202

Phone: 800.872.5327; TTY: 800.437.0833

Website: www.ed.gove/about/offices/list/osers/nidrr/index.html

About the Author

Richard Console was raised in Haddonfield, New Jersey, and attended Villanova University. Upon earning his Bachelor of Arts degree and graduating Cum Laude, he was awarded a Merit Scholarship to Rutgers University School of Law.

After receiving his degree from Rutgers, he became licensed to practice law in both New Jersey and Pennsylvania, and started his own firm. For the last fifteen years, he has been committed to protecting the rights of the injured and their families.

This book is very personal to Richard. He began advocating for brain-injured children after the two-year-old daughter of his friend, Florence suffered a brain injury and was denied coverage for hyperbaric oxygen therapy. These treatments were denied despite the fact that studies had shown marked improvements in brain injured children. Unable to afford the high cost of continuing therapy, Florence was forced to stop treatments for her daughter.

Florence's story became Richard's inspiration.

Through his research he learned that Florence was not alone—there were many other families like her that were facing the same frustrations and difficulties. In addition to committing to helping Florence get the therapy she knew would help her daughter, Richard began a pro bono project to help other families get hyperbaric oxygen therapy and other frequently denied treatments paid for by Medicaid and other insurance. In the current class action suit he is organizing, Richard is also recruiting and coordinating the work of other volunteer attorneys interested in helping families of children suffering with brain injury.

Richard focuses on the legal issues that are encountered by families of children with cerebral palsy and other brain injuries. For several years he has donated his time to various pro bono efforts, assisting these parents in getting the treatment and services their children desperately need.

Richard resides in southern New Jersey with his wife and two sons. For more information about Richard and to learn how we can help you, please visit his website at www.childbraininjury.org.